Praise for Unwinding Pain

Unwinding Pain is a remarkable story of a woman who suffered from severe total body pain for over 30 years. She has not only been free from pain since 2015, but she is also thriving and actively helping others. Her book not only tells her inspiring story but offers viable solutions. Your body knows how to heal!

—David Hanscom, MD, Orthopedic Spine Surgeon and Author of
Back in Control and *Do You Really Need Spine Surgery?*

Bonnie's book is wonderful. Using her personal healing journey, she unwinds pain step by step, using the 6 pillars of lifestyle medicine and adding her personal touch and twist. Bonnie's methods for self-care are simple, easy to follow, and actually appealing! When applied consistently, they can result in significant pain reduction or in some cases even a pain-free life.

—Sylwia P. Fowler, MD, DipABLM, Psychiatrist

This book does an excellent job of differentiating acute from chronic pain. It goes into great detail about managing chronic pain and the mind-body connection that controls pain. In each case study, she demonstrates how nonpharmacologic methods have much greater efficacy than most drugs AND have less negative side effects.

—Judith Murphy, RN, MPH, Author of
A Nurse's Journey and Observations

This book provides a road map for hope to those who've exhausted every avenue to find relief from chronic pain. Bonnie Lester shares practical tips, using the five senses and a simple tool to mark progress. This book taps into the fascinating science of neuroplasticity to change your life.

—Vickie Petz Kasper, MD, ABLM, Author of *Dressing the Wound* and Host of *Healthy Looks Great on You*

UNWINDING PAIN

Flourish Heart Press
447 Sutter St Ste 405
PMB1211
San Francisco, CA 94108

bonbonlester@gmail.com
https://www.bonnielester.com/

ISBN: 979-8-9903817-0-4 (paperback)
ISBN: 979-8-9903817-1-1 (ebook)
ISBN: 979-8-9903817-2-8 (hardcover)
ISBN: 979-8-9903817-3-5 (audiobook)

Ordering Information: Special discounts are available on quantity purchases by corporations, associations, and others. For details, email bonbonlester@gmail.com.

Publisher's Cataloging-in-Publication Data
Names: Lester, Bonnie, 1952 - .
Title: Unwinding pain : affordable and accessible ways to feel better now / Chaplain Bonnie
    Lester, M.A.
Description: San Francisco, CA : Flourish Heart Press, 2024. | Includes bibliographic references
    and index.
Identifiers: LCCN X | ISBN 9798990381711 (hardback) | ISBN
    9798990381704 (pbk) | ISBN 9798990381735 (ebook) | ISBN 9798990381728 (audiobook)
Subjects: LCSH: Pain – Treatment. | Pain – Alternative treatment. | Health behavior. | Mind and
    body therapies – Case studies. | Neuroplasticity – Case studies. | BISAC: HEALTH & FITNESS /
    Pain Management. | HEALTH & FITNESS / Healing. | MEDICAL / Alternative &
    Complementary Medicine.
Classification: LCC RB127 L47 2024 | DDC 616.0472--dc23
LC record available at https://lccn.loc.gov/X

UNWINDING PAIN

AFFORDABLE AND ACCESSIBLE WAYS
TO FEEL BETTER NOW

CHAPLAIN BONNIE LESTER, M.A.

Table of Contents

CHAPTER 1

A Mind-Blowing Event

♥

"Let me not beg for the stilling of my pain but for the heart to conquer it."
—RABINDRANATH TAGORE, POLYMATH, POET, AND PHILOSOPHER

I stood in the brightly lit examination room staring at my husband, Len. His white hair was plastered to his forehead and his face dripped with sweat. His favorite vintage shirt was inside out. He still had on old, scuffed bedroom slippers. Len had always been cool and collected, but now he sat on the exam table with a blood pressure cuff wrapped around his arm, looking confused and disoriented.

Panic swelled in my chest as I anxiously fidgeted with my wedding ring. A tall salt-and-pepper-haired male doctor knocked on the doorframe. His eyes landed on Len. He immediately approached him and removed the arm cuff and then peered at the medical chart. "So, how did this all start?"

I swallowed down my hesitancy. What had happened was really personal. I looked at Len looking at me, vulnerable and gray. He needed help, and this man was a doctor. Taking a deep breath, I told myself that the doctor had probably heard it all before.

"Well, the first sign was when Len climbed out of bed naked and stood there towering above me, confused. He kept muttering that he hadn't been here before. His eyes were wide, and he looked genuinely disoriented.

"I kept saying, 'This is our bedroom.' Len's not one to joke, and all the color had drained from his face. But I didn't see any of the classic signs of a stroke."

The doctor raised his eyebrows at that.

I continued my story, listing the signs on my fingers. "He didn't have a balance problem. He was standing straight. No slurring of speech. I gave him two aspirins for good measure, and we hurried here. The whole 14-mile drive to the hospital, he repeated the same question over and over: 'Why are we going to the hospital in Walnut Creek rather than our clinic in Pleasanton?'"

I gave a deep sigh. "It's so strange. It's like his mind is stuck on repeat. He's a brilliant software engineer who designs programs for an international business. He's never demonstrated any sign of memory loss."

The doctor reached into his jacket pocket and removed a small flashlight. He alternated the beam between Len's eyes. "What was he doing before he got out of bed?"

I blushed. "We were enjoying an afternoon session of passion."

The doctor didn't flinch at the news, and I waited for the verdict. I'd loved and depended on my husband for over 10 years. Now I found myself bracing for the diagnosis.

Scooting back and tucking the flashlight into his pocket, the doctor asked

Len to smile.

My husband's "smile" looked more like a determined grimace.

"Repeat after me: 'You can't teach old dogs new tricks,' " the doctor said.

Len's quivering voice filled the room as he repeated the exact phrase.

The doctor also tapped his fingers on Len's arms and legs and asked about the sensations he was feeling. That done, the doctor declared, "We need to send your husband for an MRI. The good news is he definitely hasn't had a stroke."

Relief poured through me. Minutes later, Len and I sat in the radiology patient section. He stared at a Hawaiian poster, then turned to me. "That looks like Sunset Beach on Oahu, where I used to surf."

At last, he was making sense. Before I could question him more about what he remembered, they called him in for his scan. I gave him a big hug, clinging to him as they ushered him away.

A half hour later, Len and I quietly talked about his memories of Hawaii, where he had been a college computer instructor. I patted his arm as he spoke. I was more at ease now that some of his mind was back and the gray color had given way to a light pale tone in his complexion.

The doctor soon found us and, looking at Len, said, "Your scan shows you have a very healthy brain, so I believe your, um, *romantic* interlude had resulted in you experiencing postcoital transient global amnesia."

For us nondoctors, what he was saying was that Len had experienced *literally* mind-blowing sex.

Mind-blowing sex? I stewed on that, having believed that was a myth.[1]

"How bad is it?" I asked, my voice cracking.

"It sounds bad, but don't worry," the doctor said, putting his pen back into his coat pocket. "Your husband's brain will reboot itself. He should regain his full faculties within the next twenty-four hours."

The doctor instructed me to keep an eye on Len for the next few days.[2] Shaking his head, he commented, "The brain is an amazing organ that can reboot itself through neuroplasticity."

I stared after the doctor with the words "reboot" and "neuroplasticity" ringing in my head.

As it turned out, the doctor was right. Within a few days, Len was back to writing complex computer programs without any trouble. The only lingering symptom he had from that day was the missing hours of memory from his time experiencing transient global amnesia.

In contrast, the memories of witnessing his mind disintegrating, and the fear of losing him, haunted me. For the past 24 years, my own existence had been overshadowed by a relentless and agonizing pain syndrome. It had left me struggling so much that my marriage to Len was my third marriage. To my dismay, my health was so bad that Len had had to step in, shouldering the burden of shopping, cooking, and laundry. The reality that he could be taken from me without notice struck me hard. I needed to become less dependent, if possible, for my own survival.

---

1   Amee Baird, "How Sex Can Literally Blow Your Mind," Psychology Today, November 14, 2019, https://www.psychologytoday.com/us/blog/sex-in-the-brain/201911/how-sex-can-literally-blow-your-mind.

2   This is pretty typical advice in transient global amnesia cases; see "Transient Global Amnesia," Mayo Clinic, August 10, 2022, https://www.mayoclinic.org/diseases-conditions/transient-global-amnesia/symptoms-causes/syc-20378531.

By telling us that our brains have the ability to reboot, the doctor had unknowingly given me a glimmer of hope for my own health. If Len's brain could reboot and get rid of amnesia, was there a possibility that I could reboot my own and get rid of my own pain?

I had to find out. I turned to YouTube and watched TED Talks that claimed I could stop my brain from sending pain messages from injuries that had healed decades before. Other videos suggested that my graduate school training on how emotions impact the body would be important in my quest. I kept searching for an explanation about neuroplasticity.

It didn't take long to find that "neuro" refers to the nervous system, which includes the brain and spinal cord. "Plasticity" comes from "*plastos,*" a Greek word meaning "moldable." Together, the words mean "moldable brain."

Through my research, I learned that I could retrain my brain's reaction to pain signals. I could actually teach my brain to be less responsive to those signals and, in doing so, experience less pain. For the first time in decades of living in almost constant agony, I had hope.

The idea of changing how the brain functioned reminded me of the physiology and psychology concepts I had learned while earning my MA in counseling and human relations.

This concept of rewiring went right back to the classic Pavlov experiment in 1904 that proved that brain reaction can be trained through repetition. Pavlov played a specific sound every time he fed the dogs food until eventually the dogs would salivate from hearing that sound without the sight and smell of food. He had in effect rewired their brains![3]

---

3   Saul McLeod, "Pavlov's Dogs Experiment and Pavlovian Conditioning Response," Simply Psychology, updated February 2, 2024, https:/www.simplypsychology.org/pavlov.html; Philippe Douyon, *Neuroplasticity: Your Brain's Superpower: Change Your Brain and Change Your Life* (Salt Lake City, UT: Izzard Ink Publishing Company, 2019), 22–25.

Armed with my new research and knowledge, I launched into my first attempt to rewire my brain. For my first step, I aimed to banish the word "pain" from my vocabulary. When I used the word "pain," my body was told to expect it and responded accordingly, but if I didn't use it, my brain was in effect being told to stop sending me these painful messages—immediately. I wanted to get on the pain-free wagon as soon as possible.

That tactic was put to the test when I woke up with my neck screaming in pain. When that thought filtered through my mind, though, I corrected it by thinking, "No, it's just tight and needs to be rubbed." Then I noticed my back was like a tightly wound spring ready to snap at any moment. Correction: my back wanted to be stretched. My left calf cramped into a torturous charley horse. Correction: my leg wanted attention, and maybe wrapping an ACE bandage around it would give it more support.

Because I wasn't thinking about the pain levels each part of my body was reporting, I didn't feel quite as bad as I normally did. My body soaked in the droplets of compassion I was offering it. I could feel it wanting more. My habit after checking in on my body was to put on a TENS unit, a machine that sends electrical nerve stimulation into the hurting area through four sticky pads to lessen the hurt. For the past 24 years, I'd placed the four electrodes on the same angry muscle groups and used the same pulsating setting to block the terrible pain in my lower back, shoulders, and neck. But not today.

Today, I rebelled against where the physical therapist had suggested that I place the electrodes and instead, I placed them in four new locations. To add to my maverick way, I daringly changed the pulsating setting. "So there, brain," I thought, "let's see if that wakes you." My surprised nerves quieted down and, to my complete shock, my pain eased a bit.

That pumped me up with exuberance that I might actually be on to something with this made-up training I was creating. I had a little perk in my step as I moved into the highlight activity of my day—walking my next-door neighbors' dog, Jingles, a black terrier.

I'd been allergic to dogs all my life, but when the magic of menopause had moved in, my allergy had checked out. So when my neighbors were going out of town and needed someone to watch their dog, I had happily volunteered. This had been the first time in my life it had been possible for me to be around the adorable, spirited creature without tears in my eyes or an itch in my throat.

When Jingles's owners had returned, I had quickly volunteered to walk her every day. Due to my health problems, this walk was often the only physical activity I could manage. A single stroll around the neighborhood would exhaust me, but I wouldn't give it up for anything. I loved that furry rescue dog. Her wagging tail and excited barks when I showed up let me know she felt the same about me.

On day one of retraining my brain, I placed a strong sugar-free mint lozenge[4] on my tongue right before knocking on Jingles's house door. Jingles barked her usual welcome. After I gave her the petting she expected, we began our walk in the chilly spring air.

Under my warm flannel shirt, I wore two fentanyl patches on my upper back. My TENS unit was clipped on my belt and set at a frequency that sent a new electrical rhythm pulsing through my muscles. I clutched my cane in my right hand to protect myself from falling when Jingles bolted after other dogs, which occurred on a daily basis.

Despite all my prep, though, pain raged through me. Slowing down, gasping,

---

4   I make sure to use sugar-free mints with xylitol, which can help promote dental health. I stay away from sorbitol because it can cause stomach upset. See Lauren Panoff, "What Is Sorbitol? Benefits, Uses, Side Effects, and More," Healthline, September 25, 2020, https://www.healthline.com/nutrition/what-is-sorbitol.

I told myself, "These are fake messages my brain is sending." I continued to walk. The misery continued. "I can't hear you," I said out loud, as though that would make my brain listen better. I took another step. "False message. False message." My muscles spasmed in my lower back, hard. "Not listening."

On all my previous walks, my thoughts had been focused on how unfair the pain was and how hard it was to move even a little bit. Today, I told myself, "Focus on the mint. What size is it?" It was shrinking, half the size of a small tooth, but it was still there. Now—ouch!—it was getting pointy and sharp. Huh, interesting; even though it was dissolving, I could still taste the mint. On and on it went like that as we progressed around the neighborhood.

The ultimate test of walking in the neighborhood came up: dog bag time. This had always been off-the-chart difficult because bending over increased the fire sensations throughout my body. On past strolls, I had always groaned on the way down. Not this time. Now, for this challenging task, I awarded myself a new lozenge. My mouth exploded with the taste of the mint. I paused for a moment with a long inhale to take in the cooling effect. The taste explosion was a blissful experience and silenced my body's usual complaints. The sensation was such a distraction that I almost forgot to dispose of the bag in a nearby receptacle.

By the end of that walk, I was exhausted, ready for a rest, but first, for my efforts I awarded myself a paper clip that I hung on a nail. I planned to hook together future earned paper clips to provide myself with a growing chain documenting my efforts at retraining my brain to dial down its false alert signals.

The Paper Clip Reward System

- Pick a healthy habit that you want to start incorporating into your life.

- Do that habit daily.

- Each time you do the habit, hook a paper clip to another paper clip.

- Hang the growing chain somewhere you can see it. This will serve as a visual representation of your progress.

As my paper clip chain grew, my homemade neuroplasticity exercises used in conjunction with scientifically based mind-body relaxation strategies were making a difference in lowering my discomfort. My goal was to use my five senses to concentrate on experiencing sensations other than burning and spasms.[5]

Within two weeks, all my activities helped me increase my walk from a half mile to a mile. Six months later, I was able to go over three miles. The longer distances became too much for sweet Jingles due to her age. This led me to search my neighborhood to find more furry critters willing to donate their enthusiasm and energy to my healing. My recruitment attempts found a frisky schnauzer and a mellow black Labrador, a recently retired diabetic alert animal.

Every day, I hit the sidewalks with my canine companions. I earned the reputation of being "the local dog walker." People thought I had a thriving pet-walking business. Instead, what I was really doing was creating a positive personal body and spirit experience.

From then on, I used self-talk and mind-body exercises throughout each day. That didn't mean I was never negative again—of course, I had my moments of despair—but I'd exercise kindness with myself to climb back on the bandwagon.

---

5   Courtney Bergart, "Using Sensory Approaches to Treat Chronic Pain," Pathways, November 11, 2019, https://www.pathways.health/blog/using-sensory-approaches-to-treat-chronic-pain/.

The reality of my life was that, in 1986, my doctors had told me that the pain I was living with was incurable,[6] but within 24 months of starting to retrain my brain, I had the miracle of experiencing 12 minutes of absolutely no burning in my neck and shoulder region. I memorized the sensation of "neutral" during those blissful 12 minutes.

Over time, the areas on my upper body that burned shrunk and the spasms in my shoulder and lower back muscles quieted. My sense of balance improved so much that I had the thrill of donating my enormous collection of fashionable canes to a senior center, and I rarely wore my TENS unit.

Despite all the improvement from dog walking, I remained on a host of medications, and with that came the horror of side effects. The worst was excessive sweating triggered by the fentanyl. I had become a sweating machine. Even on chilly days, my face was flushed and covered with perspiration. Sweat dripped down my chest and back like a constant shower. Within minutes, my clothes became soaked.

A textile specialist told me that, to avoid wet, clingy clothes, I needed to wear natural fabrics like cotton and linen that absorb sweat and keep dampness away from the body. Acrylic fabrics are like being inside a damp plastic Coke bottle. She also explained that, to stay healthy, it was important that I take care how I washed my clothes since bacteria grows in damp fabric.[7]

Another huge problem was the dry mouth side effect. My mouth was totally bone dry. I didn't have the cotton mouth that happens when you're nervous or haven't been drinking enough, but the type of dry where there's no saliva.

Whenever I had dental work, the dental hygienist always commented that

---

6   As I write this in 2024, there is a growing optimistic view that early diagnosis and treatment means my neurological pain syndrome should no longer be considered incurable.
7   Katie Crissman, "The Best Clothes for People Who Sweat Excessively," Carpe, October 1, 2020, https://mycarpe.com/blogs/sweatopedia/the-best-clothes-for-people-who-sweat-excessively.

she rarely had to suction saliva from my mouth while cleaning my teeth. My mouth's desert conditions made conversations a challenge. I had to constantly drink water to lubricate my tongue. Saliva is the shield that protects our teeth from bacteria and washes away food particles, so lacking it put my teeth at extreme risk.

The third side effect from the drugs that drove me crazy was that the medications slowed my digestion so much I became dependent on laxatives. The effective dosage changed day by day depending on the amount of opioids in my system. Never being able to fine-tune the dosage meant sometimes the laxatives caused cramps and abdominal pain.

On top of the side effects, I was also constantly worried about receiving timely refills. By the fourth week each month, I'd be counting my pills, worried they'd run out before I'd receive my new prescription. One Thanksgiving week, my refill was delayed, and I had to ration my pills. By day three, I was experiencing chills and increased burning throughout my body. By the time I received my prescription, I was at peak levels of anxiety and had intense nausea. The fear of running out was so great I'd toss and turn at night, worrying about whether I could survive without the support of fentanyl patches, Norco, and Soma.

When I was prescribed opioids, I had believed the marketing swirling around the drugs at that time. I had believed the medications would zap away the pain and give me back my life. To be honest, for a while the drugs did dial down my agony, but the burning sensations never lessened.

Despite the fact that my neuroplasticity strategies were making a difference, I viewed the strategies solely as a support to enhance the work of the opioids. That changed one windy spring day as I counted out the pills I had left for the month. I pushed the pills aside, dreaming about living without side effects and not worrying about obtaining refills. The next day, I entertained that idea again. The more I saw myself being opioid-free and side effect-free, the more

I longed to have that life.

It was then that I accepted the fact the drugs weren't getting rid of my pain, nor were they making me healthier. So in 2015, five years after the emergency room visit when I had learned so much more about the concept of neuroplasticity, I became determined to completely taper off from my pain-related medications. I contacted my wise and caring doctor, knowing how unsafe it was to do it on my own, and said, "Please get me off opioids. I'm going to rely on my mind-body practices for pain management."

Going off the powerful drugs would be difficult and challenging, both physically and emotionally. Dr. Wise-and-Caring was impressed with the progress I was making with my approach of retraining my brain, and together we devised a dosage stepping-down strategy for my six different medications.

As my medications were reduced, I went through withdrawal symptoms and experienced the pain full force. When the pain came on strong, accompanied by stomach cramps and chills, I envisioned myself living comfortably without a dry mouth, sweat pouring off my body, and dependence on laxatives. I kept telling myself that the withdrawal symptoms would be temporary; being drug-free was going to be worth it.

I'd soak in herbal baths and drink copious amounts of water and mint tea to flush the medications out of my body. Throughout each day, as the withdrawal symptoms raged through me, I would listen to uplifting music and watch my favorite documentaries.

Coming off the drugs was a ruthless marathon that included a grueling endurance test of 48 straight hours of insomnia. Every muscle screamed and time seemed to stand still as I withered in pain. I managed to put on meditation tapes and tried to visualize how I'd feel once the chemicals were out of my body. When sleep finally came, though, the withdrawal experience faded. I was well on my way to living life without opioids.

Each person's experience with opioids is unique. It's important to remember that tapering off is not something that should be attempted all at once or without the counsel of a medical professional to ensure your safety through this huge undertaking.

After 10 months, I was able to completely taper off all six drugs. Like Alice falling into Wonderland, I was now moving into a new, vibrant reality without fentanyl patches on my back and the other opioids that had drained the vitality out of my body. Now, free of the drugs' clutches, my health suddenly came back to me. No longer did my neck, arms, and back feel like they were burning. I was steady on my feet without back spasms tugging at me. Best of all, I could now sit comfortably for hours at a time.

The neuroplasticity training and all my mind-body exercises had paid off. I didn't recover the 33-year-old body I had had before I developed my neuro-logical pain syndrome, but I was now a pain-free 63-year-old with growing vitality and passion to get on with life.

I celebrated the pain-free version of myself by volunteering my chaplaincy services to the owner of my schnauzer dog-walking companion. The dog's owner needed a transplant. While he and his wife were awaiting notification that it was time to travel to a national transplant hospital in New Orleans, I suggested that I come with them to provide emotional and spiritual support while they were at the hospital. As soon as they received word that it was time to head to New Orleans, I packed my bag to catch the next flight out.

As I readied to leave for the airport, I was overcome with thoughts of my past personal health challenges. I couldn't believe that the woman who had struggled to even move or perform daily tasks was now getting on a plane to be of deep service to those in a time of need.

I wouldn't have ever been able to do this without my first dog-walking companion, Jingles. She had given me the ability to take the first few steps in my healing adventure. Those first months had been so shaky, but her presence had kept me going. On the way to the airport, I stopped by her house to celebrate the healing those steps had led me to. As I said goodbye to my sweet pal, Len captured that moment in a picture, which now hangs in a place of honor in our living room.

This book shares the proven strategies and techniques I used to train my brain and improve my overall quality of life. Not only have they worked for me, but they have also helped countless people living with back injuries, fibromyalgia, complex regional pain syndrome (CRPS), autoimmune diseases, post-stroke pain, osteoarthritis, and many other diseases.

The amazing thing about what I discovered is that a high percentage of people living with chronic pain who take a disciplined approach in practicing these whole-person strategies can achieve an enhancement in their overall well-being in only a few weeks.

Most people report consistently feeling better when they regularly incorporate the changes into their daily lives. When I began my journey, I was aiming for "a lot better." Not everyone improves beyond their hopes and dreams, but they can experience an improvement in their day-to-day life and also manage flare-ups and setbacks.

My hope for you as you read this book is that you will feel empowered to take control of your health. In doing so, you will incorporate customized self-care activities that will not only unwind your pain but also improve your overall health.

REMEMBER:

- Neuroplasticity is the brain's natural ability to reboot itself.
- Self-care of chronic pain can bring relief.
- Home-based pain management strategies work.

CHAPTER 2

The Origin of My Pain

♥

"It can't be done for you; it must be done by you."

—FRANK SONNENBERG, AUTHOR

I sat in my Nissan Sentra, waiting for the stopped traffic to budge. It was a Friday in 1986, and I was on the main street in Larkspur, California. The soft sounds of news rattled from the radio. My mind grappled with work pressures, trying to figure out how to navigate the newest office politics.

A deafening roar sounded behind me. Before I could look in my rearview mirror, my head forcefully thrust forward then backward as if I were a lifeless Raggedy Ann doll. Searing pain shot up and down my spine, especially on the left side of my neck where the seatbelt forced me back into the seat.

A drunk driver in a BMW sedan going 45 miles an hour had plowed straight into my back bumper. The impact transformed my car into a crumpled accordion, while the BMW merely had a crinkled front hood with steam hissing from its engine.

"What fresh hell is this?" I wondered. Flaring pain rose along my spine and up my neck, plus my ears rang. Four years post-surgery for a herniated disc resulting from a healthy nine-pound baby, I was just barely starting to feel normal. Now here I was, in shock and smarting from new pain.

After the accident, I headed to the emergency room to get checked out and was saddled with a bulky neck brace and a pile of prescriptions for muscle spasms and discomfort. On Monday, after popping two Tylenol, I returned to work at Mill Valley's recreation department. Our mission was to give the local residents the opportunity to improve their quality of life by offering health and wellness classes and providing social events. All of this was intended to encourage active lifestyles in the community.

Since the accident, I had hardly been able to move, and I definitely couldn't sleep. Despite how bad I felt, I dragged myself to my office desk carrying a bulky laptop and back support pillow. Wincing in pain, I set up my laptop and briefly explained my condition to my concerned coworkers.

As I tried to dive into my computer work, I discovered that my dominant left hand had gone numb and lacked the strength and coordination to hit the right keys. I ended up adopting the tediously slow method of typing with only my right hand. Pain screamed through my body and grew louder with each passing minute. I fought back tears, knowing my supervisor would soon notice me falling behind on my workload and would voice her frustration that I was missing a deadline.

By lunchtime, I called my doctor, who recommended going on short-term disability. Seeing no other choice, I reluctantly did so. Over the weeks that followed, my pain rapidly increased. The baffled doctor played hot potato and passed me on to an orthopedist.

Within a week, my tall, well-built, curly red-haired orthopedist was flipping through my patient history. "You suffered a brachial plexus injury," he finally said.

I wrinkled my nose. "Brachial what?"

"It's an injury to the nerves responsible for sending signals from your spinal cord to your shoulders, arms, and hands. These particular nerves are critical for control of muscle function and relaying information to the brain.

"This type of nerve damage is common in car accidents, especially when the body experiences intense jolting movements, like what happened when your car was rear-ended. You may experience weakness, loss of muscle control, and intense pain in your arms."

He sounded confident that rest would help, and he prescribed two additional medications to see if that would quiet down my symptoms. Four months later, the red-headed orthopedist declared that my scans and neurological tests were inconclusive. Since I should have recovered from my accident by that point, he also played hot potato and referred me to a pain clinic for therapy.

The clinic's physical therapy appointments included light massage and heat treatments that temporarily eased the spasms but did nothing to heal my condition. It's important to note that clinics in 1986 were nothing like the pain clinics today that offer pain treatment modalities like acupuncture, biofeedback, chiropractic care, cognitive behavioral therapy, dietary advice, and a wide variety of deep tissue and lymphatic massage.

Months dragged by. My days filled with physical therapy appointments followed by short walks and then reclining on the sofa with a heating pad soothing the ache. My meals were based on units of pain—anything requiring a can opener was out due to the pain in my hand. Ditto for holding a knife to spread a nut butter. That meant that for lunch I'd slap slices of turkey between two pieces of bread after I took my noontime dose of anti-inflammatories and muscle relaxants. School day afternoons found me ignoring my body's complaints as I headed to my son's favorite specialty sandwich shops for his after-school snack. I hoped these treats would make up for the fact I couldn't do all the fun parenting activities I had envisioned myself doing with him. The weekends were more of the same survival tactics.

One day, as I painfully shuffled around my neighborhood, my left hand and arm felt like I had a sunlamp beaming its hot rays on them. I hadn't gotten a sunburn, nor had I burned myself cooking. The sensation subsided but then returned with a vengeance the next day. This same sensation also happened on the left side of my neck for a couple of hours before it stopped suddenly.

From that day on, my body started playing games with me. Randomly, it'd zap me with flaming hot heat like I had been lit on fire. I would yelp and try to cool off, but nothing worked. Then, with no apparent reason, the burn would stop.

I would experiment to get my body to reveal what instigated the burning. One day I'd wear long sleeves. I'd flare up like a bonfire. The next day, still wearing long sleeves, nothing would happen. I'd do the same with short sleeves. I'd play with the temperature in the house—random results. I tracked when it happened. My body would burst into heat morning, noon, night, and in the wee hours of the morning. I even tracked what kind of food I ate, but no secret code revealed itself.

On a grocery store trip, I noticed that the sensations increased in the frozen food section, especially when I was reaching for the frozen vegetables. That was my first clue that I was hypersensitive to temperatures and drafts (or my body was telling me it really didn't like frozen peas!). This led me to start wrapping my left arm and hand with an ACE bandage to protect them from fluctuating temperatures—and to protect the rest of me from being hit with extreme internal temperatures. That quieted the burning down a little bit.

My body still liked playing games, though. It had a special connection with the fog and rain. Whenever fog or rain rolled in off the Northern California coast, my hand would swell, throb, and turn bright red. To me, it felt like my arm and hand were on fire, but when someone else touched them, to them they felt ice cold.[8]

This led me back to Dr. Redhead's office. He sighed. "I was hoping I wouldn't have to tell you this, but all your symptoms point to the neurological condition known as reflex sympathetic dystrophy."

In the 1990s, reflex sympathetic dystrophy, or RSD, underwent a name change, and it's now known as complex regional pain syndrome (CRPS). There is published evidence of this condition that dates back to the Civil War, specifically after the Battle of Gettysburg. During that time, an army doctor, Dr. S. Weir Mitchell, created a specialty ward to treat injured soldiers suffering from "neural maladies" (in 21st century terms, "conditions that affect the nervous system"). While treating the soldiers, he observed that some of them experienced persistent regions of burning pain that continued long after their battle wounds had healed. He was the first to describe CRPS and publish his findings.[9]

Dr. Redhead informed me that even though 122 years had passed since the Civil War, there was still no cure for CRPS, and no medication effectively got rid of the burning. He warned me that it would take courage to live with this condition.

My bleak prognosis motivated me to initiate an international search for treatment. The search didn't yield any promising curative treatments in the U.S. or abroad. I found an ominous prognosis among the neurology diagnostic and treatment textbooks. In the vast majority of CRPS cases, the condition

---

8   David Kloth, Andrea Trescot, and Francis Riegler, *Pain-Wise: A Patient's Guide to Pain Management* (Hobart, NY: Hatherleigh Press, 2011), 89.
9   S. Weir Mitchell, George R. Morehouse, and William Keen, *Gunshot Wounds and Other Injuries of Nerves* (Philadelphia, PA: J.B. Lippincott & Co., 1864).

led to one or more of the following:

- institutionalization

- divorce

- suicide (the suicide rate among CRPS patients is so high that the condition is referred to as the "suicide disease"[10])

The grim forecast made me very afraid. My son was so young and needed his mom. I wasn't going to be taken from him because of this condition. That wasn't a price I was willing to pay. Right then and there, I vowed to do whatever I could to see him go to college one day.

Dr. Redhead referred me to an anesthesiologist who was experimenting with the use of stellate ganglion nerve blocks for pain management. This involved injecting local anesthetic into the bundle of nerves near my collarbone. The hoped-for outcome was that the injection would not only numb the sympathetic nerves in my neck region but also permanently turn off the pain signals from the accident.

The first time I underwent the block, I was ecstatic to discover I no longer felt like I was burning up. But 36 hours later, I was engulfed by a wave of scorching pain that stayed with me until the next treatment. This was the pattern for the subsequent four nerve blocks. Each time the block wore off, I sunk into a deep valley of despair.

When I voiced my frustrations, the anesthesiologist put a positive spin on my situation. "Your temporary improvement means you're a good candidate for a surgical nerve block called a sympathectomy that's being done by surgeons affiliated with a prestigious medical school's pain clinic. The procedure creates a permanent nerve block by removing a portion of your sympathetic

---

10   James Doulgeris, "CRPS, a New Four-Letter Word from Hell," Reflex Sympathetic Dystrophy Syndrome Association, June 5, 2019, https://rsds.org/anewfourletterword/.

nerve chain that runs along your spine. You'll no longer experience CRPS symptoms."

The promise of being CRPS symptom–free filled me with hope that at last I could be out of pain and able to do things that for so long I hadn't been able to do. I looked forward to being able to participate in my son's field trips around the Bay Area and accompanying my husband on his annual treks to his favorite sporting events.

The morning of the surgery, my tall surgeon loomed over me as he came to greet me. His nicotine-stained fingers reached down to touch my left hand as he said, "Your ice-cold hand and the internal burning you're experiencing are going to disappear forever."

After the surgery, I was shocked to discover that the surgery had made my condition worse. My burning regions had spread throughout my body, and my dominant hand still felt ice cold to others. But, to make things worse, I could no longer grasp or hold anything. It would take 26 years of arm and hand exercises for me to recover the ability to hold a regular fork, handwrite letters, and type with both hands.

As I adjusted to my reduced abilities, my husband was promoted to the first of many positions that required relocating to other states. With my eight-year-old son in tow, I navigated our first major move from the San Francisco Bay Area to Reno, Nevada, without the use of my dominant hand and with burning sensations on the entire left side of my body. (Interesting side note: Though I moved several more times after that point, none of the locations I resided in reduced my pain.)

My doctors labeled my status "permanent and stationary," meaning I would not improve. Despite that incredibly bleak diagnosis, whenever the family moved, I immediately worked to build a relationship with a local physician to keep my condition as stable as possible. With each move, I secretly hoped a new physician would offer a treatment that would help—if not heal—my CRPS. But the doctors seemed to be better at talking about how my condition was identified during the Civil War than they were at bringing me any healing.

Every new city increased my feelings of isolation as I realized that, soon enough, we would be moving again. My husband worked long hours and traveled extensively. My son attended school and tried to adjust to the constant changes that came with moving, and he flew to California to stay with his dad every summer and on major holidays.

A wave of despair engulfed me when my son departed for his first holiday trip. After wiping away my tears at the airport, I traveled home. I sat in the empty house waiting for his call that he'd arrived and connected with his dad. I told myself that he was going to have a great time with his dad and stepmother. He always had in the past, so there was no need to worry. And besides that, he was going to get to spend time with my mom. He'd always loved spending time with his loving, spunky grandmother. This was going to be a cherished memory for him.

Just thinking of my mom snapped me into shape. If she knew I was throwing a pity party for myself, she'd recite her famous motto, "Pull yourself together and get on with living." Thinking about her motto filled me with the determination to apply a resilient mindset to being away from my son. I wanted to wake up by greeting the morning sun and to end the day by smiling at the evening moon. To do those things, I needed to figure out how to keep a spark in my life.

By that point, I was using my paper clip reward system (chapter 1) every day to help me do the exercises my physical therapist had prescribed. Now I wanted to create strategies to improve my mood. The challenge facing me was battling the dread I had when I woke up every morning. I figured the best way to do that would be to find something to get excited about each day so I'd stop mulling over my CRPS.

As I thought about my current situation, I recalled my college studies of the four pillars for general well-being: physical, mental, social, and spiritual. (In chapter 9, you'll see that these pillars evolved over the years from four pillars to six.) The idea that positive lifestyle changes could improve overall health excited me and was something I wanted to explore. I figured that enhancing those four dimensions of my life could possibly pave a healing path before me, and I was excited to find out what would happen.

REMEMBER:

- Doctors can't feel your pain.

- Creating a more comfortable life requires you to take an active role in your treatment activities.

- Even in adversity, there's an opportunity to experience less pain.

CHAPTER 3

Courage, Resilience, and Transformation

♥

"Sometimes the smallest step in the right direction ends up being the biggest step in your life. Tiptoe if you must, but take a step."

—NAEEM CALLAWAY, AUTHOR

In my quest to fully integrate the four pillars of health into my life, the need to begin nurturing my emotional health became starkly clear. The pain and limitations of my health had pressed so hard on me that I struggled to get through each day. I longed to live life full of purpose again.

I grabbed a pen in my nondominant hand and jotted down ideas about how I could unlock my potential.

I worked on putting together the different elements into a curriculum, as I had done in my former job. As I dove in, working on this for the next few days, a full blueprint emerged, one that I proudly called AIM—an acronym for Affirmation, Image, and Management.

♥

If you aim higher than you expect, you can reach higher than you dreamed of.
—RICHARD BRANSON, ENTREPRENEUR

The essence of AIM is to elevate the emotional well-being of those suffering from pain by putting more purpose and passion into their lives. The foundation of the program is built on the finding that balancing your emotional health has a powerful positive impact on your physical condition.[11] By incorporating this, you're addressing yourself as a whole person, not just addressing your physical symptoms.

From those days of sitting down and filling out the blueprint, I applied the program in my life and refined the steps as I worked through them. When the program started improving my life, including reducing my pain, I started teaching it to others.

The program is forged from personal experience and tested through my own challenges and my work with hundreds of clients. Over the years, I have witnessed amazing results. I'm confident that if you try the program out in your own life, your days will be a little bit better.

AIM's Three Core Principles

Principle 1: Affirmation (A)

Research found that individuals with a strong sense of purpose experience better overall physical and mental health.[12] Knowing this, I started each

---

11   Jennifer Robinson, "How Does Mental Health Affect Physical Health?" WebMD, September 23, 2023, https://www.webmd.com/mental-health/how-does-mental-health-affect-physical-health.

12   Bernes-Zare Illene, "The Importance of Having a Sense of Purpose," Psychology Today, June 4, 2019, https://www.psychologytoday.com/us/blog/flourish-and-thrive/201906/the-importance-having-sense-purpose.

day with an affirmation that made me feel optimistic about myself: "I have purpose and I matter."

It wasn't enough to mutter it. I had to embody it and believe it. At first, doing that was extremely hard since the affirmation seemed contradictory. I could barely move. How could I have a purpose?

Working with my doubts, I would whisper, "Bonnie, you have purpose. You do. It might not seem like it right now, but it's here. You have to find it. And you do matter. You know you matter. Let that in."

Principle 2: Image (I)

Our choice of clothes affects our mindset and our mood. Jennifer Dragonette, a psychologist at the Newport Institute in California, commented that our clothes choices that might seem "insignificant can actually lead to dwindling motivation and productivity."[13] Getting out of PJs and sweats, especially when in pain, can shift our focus from inactivity to purposeful action and give us a boost against feeling defeated.

Principle 3: Management (M)

Who says management is all spreadsheets and fancy suits? Well, surprise. We're all managers, even if your LinkedIn profile doesn't say "Executive Manager of XYZ Company." Management extends beyond professional hierarchies. When you make sure there's food in the fridge and something to eat at dinnertime, you're a manager. You might not be the big CEO in charge of hundreds of people, but you're still the CEO of your own life.

In addition to the three principles of the AIM program, over time it became

---

13   Lindsay Champion, "What Happens When You Wear PJs All Day, According to a Psychologist," PureWow, June 1, 2020, https://www.purewow.com/fashion/wearing-pajamas.

clear I needed to add other self-care practices to support a fuller life. No, I am not talking about bubble baths. I'm talking about taking care of yourself.

As a result, I added the ABCs of Life Enrichment Principles to the program.

A. **Explore Your Negative Landmines:** Identify what diminishes your well-being. What are those things that chip away from your ability to feel your best? Maybe it feels like your opinion no longer matters, or like people around you are enjoying a life in living color while you're sidelined to black and white. Or maybe you feel like you're under a life sentence of pain. Uncovering these "happiness stealers" is crucial.

B. **Understand How Pain Negatively Impacts You:** Identify the pitfalls in your current life. What is currently bringing you down? Maybe your social life has evaporated? Or maybe your family has been impacted negatively? Or maybe the thing that's really getting to you is the condition of your house, which you don't have the strength to organize. Chronic pain can be a brutal taskmaster that steals our focus, attention, and quality of life if we aren't careful. But the good news is you have the power to be your own superhero.

C. **Build Your Program:** To counter that attack you've been under, it's time to add more positive things back into your life. If you don't know what to do, a good place to start is to list things you wish you could do. The top of my list, besides being with my parrots, included researching 18th- and 19th-century medicine and being of service to others.

For you, maybe you always wanted to speak French. Or are you curious about art history? Or do you want to refinish furniture? You'll find that engaging in an activity you find fulfilling improves all areas of your life. Don't immediately rule things out. You'll be surprised how a touch of ingenuity can make things you thought you couldn't do work.

My Journey Through the AIM Program

For my AIM program, I created hour-long weekly pro bono community workshops to help other people suffering from health challenges, family life challenges, or both. This was the perfect answer for me to be of service and build local connections—my two must-haves for happiness.

Depending on where I was living at the time, I offered these weekly workshops in Reno, Atlanta, and then back in the San Francisco Bay Area. Producing these programs took passion and a whole lot of determination. I had to cope with the fact that I was limited to one-handed, focused, short bursts of computer work. Sitting for hours in front of a computer wasn't an option.

Speech-to-text software had just come out, and I took it for a test drive, finding that it took all my wisdom and transformed it into gibberish on the screen. That being a no go, I resorted to using a large tablet balanced on an easel and drew graphs and diagrams. Well, correction, I *tried* to draw graphs and diagrams, but since I was using my nondominant hand, the images were funny squiggles and abstract art. Amazingly, I still managed to get my points across, and I got a lot of good-natured laughs from the audience. Score one for Team Ambidexterity.

Over the years, I noticed that my pain would dial down when I stood in front of my eager students. I'd feel a sense of joy as I watched them jot down my ideas and answered their questions. Okay, I admit it, I was blown away by the enthusiastic thank-yous and positive responses, too.

But then the landmark year of 2015 happened. That's when I kicked CRPS to the curb, extinguished the fire in my body, and reclaimed the use of my left hand. The impossible had happened. My success in my healing journey came down to me working with my brain using scientific principles I had uncovered from researchers.

In the turbulent year of 2020, when the world turned topsy-turvy, my AIM workshops took a bold leap into the virtual realm. Say hello to my pandemic-inspired individualized Zoom classes.

At the age of 68, I'd been pain-free for five years. To celebrate, I purchased a laptop with a great camera and entered the Zoomosphere.

I anxiously digested all the best practices for using Zoom, like making sure to unmute myself so clients could hear me. Then I sucked up all the courage I could muster and sent out Zoom invitations to one of my workshops. I felt like I had climbed onto a magic carpet that was now whisking me to distant lands to show people how they could improve their health and spirits.

I offered up my classes on busting insurmountable pain to my social media followers. When registrations from all over the U.S., Canada, the U.K., and the Netherlands poured in faster than you can say "public health crisis," I was so shocked my mind spun. I felt like a daytime TV talk show anchor. I soon found myself hosting so many international one-on-one meetings that I tucked a time zones cheat sheet near my computer to keep everything straight.

The results from the classes and people following the program filled me with joy and awe.

- One beautiful lady overcame her depression and volunteered to drive people to medical appointments.

- Another lady was so inspired that she decided to shake off her inertia and organize weekly outdoor social events for her senior condo complex.

- A man became inspired to do online coaching sessions to help small business owners navigate websites so they could apply for pandemic-related funding.

- A bedridden client with intense flare-ups became a successful virtual assistant.

- An older man with severe arthritis found a new calling as a remote mentor, guiding future computer programmers.

- Another client spent her flare-up downtime touring international museums on YouTube and used the information for later presentations at regional senior centers.

The AIM program even helped a personal friend with terminal cancer, who used the program to bring himself emotional comfort in his final months. He was known for his skills at rehabilitating wildlife that had been injured in urban settings. As his health declined, the program inspired him to achieve a long-held dream.

He and his friends gathered his extensive vinyl record collection. They launched an online auction that drew attention from vinyl collectors around the world. The income from the sale of his collection enabled him to form a wildlife conservation charity. Seeing his dream materialize buoyed his spirits, even though he was in the last weeks of his life. At the time of his passing, his organization was actively saving the lives of animals.

Throughout this book, I'll be introducing you to some of my clients who improved their overall health by practicing science-based life-improving strategies. I invite you not to just read the stories, but to also see what you can integrate into your own life to help you on your healing journey.

Case Study: Lupus

After regaining the use of my dominant hand, I discovered the joy of designing spiritual jewelry. I started to create pieces for women with health challenges and eventually posted them on Instagram. Lynn reached out to me to purchase a handcrafted amethyst necklace for her new off-the-shoulder lavender Christmas gown. Amethyst's purple is the color used to raise awareness for lupus. Lynn reached out again after reading my Instagram posts about reducing pain if you have autoimmune diseases and chronic pain. She wanted to talk about her lupus flare-ups.

Lupus

Lupus is a notorious troublemaker. This sneaky autoimmune disease affects approximately five million people worldwide, wreaking havoc on their immune systems.[14] It attacks healthy cells in tissues and organs with antibodies that cause inflammation and tissue damage, leading to rashes and skin ulcers. The assault also goes after joints, kidneys, skin, blood cells, lungs, and the heart. If that's not challenging enough, lupus sometimes attacks the brain, leading to headaches and cognitive difficulties.

Lupus has a soft spot for going after women between 15 and 44. This group makes up 90% of lupus cases.[15] People aren't born with the disease, but genetics can tip them toward getting it. Scientists haven't cracked the code for a cure, but there are ways to wrestle the symptoms to be more under control.[16]

Symptoms[17]

- Muscle and joint pain
- Fever
- Rashes
- Chest pain

- Hair loss
- Sun or light sensitivity
- Kidney problems

---

14 "Lupus Facts and Statistics," Lupus Foundation of America, last updated July 23, 2021, https://www.lupus.org/resources/lupus-facts-and-statistics.
15 "Lupus Facts and Statistics."
16 Elizabeth Zimmerman, "Science Saturday: Lupus Rates Increasing, Communities of Color Especially Vulnerable," Mayo Clinic News Network, July 23, 2022, https://newsnetwork.mayoclinic.org/discussion/science-saturday-lupus-rates-increasing-communities-of-color-especially-vulnerable/.
17 M. Cojocaru et al., "Manifestations of Systemic Lupus Erythematosus," *Maedica: A Journal of Clinical Medicine* 6, no. 4 (2011): 330–36.

- Mouth sores
- Prolonged or extreme fatigue
- Anemia

- Memory problems
- Blood clotting
- Eye disease

Risk Factors[18]

- More common in women
- Most often diagnosed between the ages of 15 and 45
- More common in African Americans, Hispanics, and Asian Americans

Diagnosis

- Laboratory tests, including complete blood count, erythrocyte sedimentation rate, kidney and liver assessment, urinalysis, and antinuclear antibody test
- Imaging tests such as a chest x-ray or echocardiogram
- Kidney or skin biopsy

Common Triggers

- Sun exposure
- Stress
- Fatigue
- Discontinuation of lupus medications[19]

18 "Lupus," MayoClinic.org, October 21, 2022. https://www.mayoclinic.org/diseases-conditions/lupus/symptoms-causes/syc-20365789

19 Lupus Foundation of Northern California, "What Are Common Triggers for Lupus Flares?" September 7, 2020, YouTube video, 3:36, https://youtu.be/jhHSGDUC258?si=Y7xN6FlF5D3tB2CO.

Treatments

- Nonsteroidal anti-inflammatory drugs (NSAIDs)

- Corticosteroids

- Antimalarial drugs

- Immunosuppressants

- Biological therapies

- Lifestyle modification: exercise, diet, stress management, rest, and sleep

- Sun protection, including sunscreen and protective clothes

When Lynn came into view on the computer screen that sunny April afternoon, she sat in front of her apartment's windows. They soared from floor to ceiling, giving a view of downtown Toronto's skyline and the giant CN Tower in the background.

Lynn wore her amethyst jewelry with a silky green flowing blouse, and her trendy platinum pixie cut hairstyle accentuated her full moon–shaped face—a side effect of prednisone, a common lupus medication. In the pre-pandemic era, Lynn had loved living on the 20th floor of her high-rise apartment.

However, COVID had transformed her excitement into anxiety. Fearful of catching COVID, she worried about stepping into the small elevator with other potential virus-carrying passengers due to her compromised immune system. The fact everyone wore masks only calmed her nerves somewhat. She knew the possibility of touching the wrong thing or breathing in the virus was a huge risk to her health. Every time she stepped into the elevator, her increased stress levels aggravated her lupus pain symptoms.

Amidst our greeting, the bark of a dog caught my attention, prompting me to ask for a doggy introduction. Lynn pulled up a fluffy white powder puff dog. "This is Cynthia."

The miniature poodle stared into the camera. Her big brown eyes peeped up at me through the wild curly hair. She licked Lynn's face, then settled comfortably in her lap. Her loving nature won me over instantly, and so did all those adorable corkscrew white curls.

Lynn told me that when she was a college student, she had frequent headaches and achy joints. The condition had gotten so bad she had visited the student health center. As she checked in, a pamphlet on autoimmune diseases caught her eye. Leafing through it, a sense of dread settled over her when she saw an unmistakable butterfly-shaped rash adorning the face of a patient, mirroring the peculiar pattern of eruptions she had dismissed as stress-induced acne in the prior weeks.

When she told the doctor about the connection she had made, he put her through tests confirming she had lupus. During the early years of her diagnosis, she was able to keep the flare-ups under control with medications. Life marched on and she married and launched a successful career. Then she became pregnant, which was considered high risk for a lupus patient. Through close monitoring, she was able to give birth to a healthy daughter.

Unfortunately, her post-pregnancy life, with the challenges of child-raising and a high-pressure financial career, brought on a rough patch with lupus. She coped with it the best she could and kept plowing through over the years. She was able to help her daughter graduate from high school.

But the disease took a toll on her relationship with her husband. He finally opted to end their 25-year marriage. Chronic illness is often a big factor in divorce.[20]

---

20 "Divorce Rates Are Higher When the Wife Is Ill," Hecht & Associates, May 17, 2022, https://www.hechtassociates.com/blog/2022/05/divorce-rates-are-higher-when-the-wife-is-ill/.

A year after Lynn's divorce, at the age of 54, she began dating a dog lover like herself, but after COVID hit, she rarely saw him. All her focus turned to keeping her business afloat. As she soldiered on, her joints shouted louder.

After hearing her backstory, I asked, "Did you know that we can reprogram our brains to help us feel better?"

She stroked Cynthia's groomed coat. "Okay, how?"

"Right now, your shoulders are relaxed as your brain responds to being with your dog. I can teach you to do more things like that, so your brain will calm more often and you'll feel better."

She peered at me. "My colleagues used to have respect for me and were impressed with the deals I closed. Now, I feel like they're writing me off the longer I go without bringing in new accounts. I'm half the person I used to be."

I flinched with the sting of that statement, knowing her pain all too well. "When you have a calm brain, you'll have the emotional energy to do what you need to for your business. Plus, I can help you discover ways to quiet the aches."

She placed Cynthia on the floor and picked up her pen to take notes.

"I suggest you implement my simple three-step AIM program designed to work with your pain."

"Consider me on board," she said quickly.

"Great. The first step is choosing your personal affirmation and repeating it aloud every morning as soon as you wake up."

She picked up her phone and scrolled through it, mumbling something about a special list.

She read the affirmation, "I believe in myself and, though I may have obstacles in my way, I can choose to continue on my path because it leads to my goals."

I gave her a thumbs up. "Perfect!"

She read it over again. "It is, isn't it?"

"Print it out and hang it on your bedroom wall to say daily."

She reached down to gather up Cynthia for more cuddles as we moved on to step two.

"You look lovely and professional, but I want to make sure that you understand that dressing up the way that you're currently doing has a huge impact on improving your frame of mind. You want to dress well for the day and avoid staying in PJs all day."

She gave a guilty laugh, like I had busted her. "Since I started working remotely, I rarely wear daytime clothes. I only change out of my robe to buy groceries once a week, to walk Cynthia, and when I have Zoom meetings."

"You and the rest of the world," I said, then shared, "When I shifted out of baggy sweats and learned from YouTube fashion videos about how to put together an inexpensive, comfortable daytime wardrobe, my outlook improved."

"Fine. Dressing up, here I come."

That covered, we talked about step three, management. I explained that this was her opportunity to explore how her current situation impacted her emotional well-being and then pivot to doing things that help her smile on her darkest days.

She answered easily: time with her dog, daughter, and significant other.

"Great. Let's keep those in mind and create a program that speaks to you. What do you most enjoy doing?"

Lynn crossed her arms, being careful not to bump the dog snoring on her lap. "Work with numbers and keep Cynthia close by."

As I watched the bond between her and her dog, I suddenly had an idea. "Did you know that service dogs help people with health issues enter the work and educational environment, but the cost of training them is steep?"

Her forehead crinkled in concern. "That's not good at all." She stroked her dog. "I can't imagine what I would've done without the comfort of Cynthia." She sighed, still stewing over that fact. "That's a tragedy."

The next time we met, she smiled brightly. She jumped in and immediately told me that she was starting a foundation that offered grants to pay for dogs to be trained as service dogs to give more people access to trained animals.

On our last call, when Lynn and Cynthia came into view, I saw not only a smiling dog owner and a happy dog wagging her tail, but also multiple pictures of service dogs taped onto the side window frames. These dogs were trained to help people with diabetes, epilepsy, PTSD, and autism.

Lynn's picture gallery was to keep her inspired in launching her foundation. Lynn had found a way to combine her love for numbers and her appreciation for dogs into a program. Her aches did decrease and, most importantly, she was able to reclaim her former dynamic business abilities.

She reported that she now steps into the elevator excited to greet her neighbors and seize the chance to share information about her new service dog foundation.

As we said our final goodbye, she laughed and said, "AIM's step two led me to view fashion advice shows on YouTube. I discovered I'm an inverted strawberry, which means my shoulders are wider than my hips. I'm supposed to stay away from puff-sleeved tops and wear figure-flattering V-neck outfits instead. After I'm done repeating my morning affirmation, I put on my fashionable day wear and feel good about myself."

Lynn and I are just two examples of how my AIM program enriches lives despite discomfort. The best part of AIM is that it is a home-based program that can enhance your "between medical appointments" life.

Too often, a person living with chronic pain finds their life consumed by medical and therapy appointments. By incorporating the three simple steps of AIM, you'll be reclaiming an identity other than that of a pain sufferer.

In the next chapter, you'll learn why pain persists in your life and how to say no to it. This will be a game changer.

REMEMBER:

- You can redefine yourself despite your pain.

- You can achieve your goals.

- You can feel good about yourself.

- You can experience happiness and fulfillment, no matter your health condition.

CHAPTER 4

Unravel the Mystery of Pain

♥

"[Humanity's] greatest evil is to suffer pain."
—SAINT THOMAS AQUINAS

Let's say it typically takes you half an hour to complete a short crossword puzzle. How much time do you think it would take if you received constant electrical shocks to your hands? Perhaps you think it would take much longer because the shocks would distract you from your task.

Many people would be distracted by the pain and take longer to complete the task. Other people would use the task to distract themselves from the sensations. By using focus techniques, they would work more efficiently. Still others would be able to avoid thinking about the discomfort and stay on task, but the energy required to ignore the unpleasant sensations would rob them of the usual pleasure they get from completing a crossword puzzle.

How can people who are subjected to the same type of pain experience it so differently?

To unlock this mystery, we must explore the nature of pain. I know you're not interested in earning a PhD in physiology, so I'm going to provide you with a basic overview of how your body and brain process pain. By understanding the dynamics behind the pain messages, you'll see that there are steps you can take to lower their volume.

The Physiology of Pain and House Alarms

It may surprise you to hear that pain is generated by our brains, not by our damaged body parts. Our brains and our spinal columns make up the central nervous system (CNS). This system carries information from our nerve fibers, which detect conditions that are potentially threatening to our bodies, such as extreme temperatures, injuries, and other body stressors.

When the CNS senses danger, it then acts by sending warning messages to the brain that trouble is brewing. It's your body's Morse code that works when you absentmindedly grab for a hot casserole dish without using an oven mitt. When these sensors in your hand feel the heat, they instantly send a danger signal to your brain, and you immediately withdraw your unprotected hand.

Your brain's decoding work involves assessing how loud an alarm it should be generating. Sometimes its alarms blare like a bugle; other times, they're like a gentle ripple. The intensity of the alarms sent can be louder if you're experiencing fear, anxiety, depression, or fatigue. And if you have a history of pain, that affects how your brain processes new pain. Basically, if you've ever previously experienced pain, your prize is that any future pain alarms may be exaggerated. This is because your brain has learned from your past that louder alarms get your attention.

The Two Faces of Pain

There are two types of pain. It's important to know the difference since the treatment is different for each.

The pain from the hot casserole dish is acute pain. Compare this pain to an older brother who will do anything to grab your attention and notify your body to quickly respond. The best way to react to this kind of pain is to rest and protect the wounded area. This type of pain lasts from the time of injury to when the tissues have healed. This normally takes no more than three months.

Unfortunately, the big brother acute pain has an annoying little sister called chronic or persistent pain. The little sister seems to be constantly nagging for attention. She might show up after her big brother fades away after three months. She's good at using spasms, cramping, tingling, burning, and other unpleasant sensations to get and keep the attention she craves. She'll do this for however long she can get away with it. Her antics often impact work, social life, and family relations. Having her nipping at you can lead to trouble sleeping, anxiety, and depression, which amplify her agonizing sensations.

Taming your little sister's antics is a challenge. In the past, physicians often believed that patients whose suffering existed after their pathology had healed were either experiencing mental health problems or seeking financial compensation or drugs.[21] This is because the medical field at the time lacked the understanding of the connection between the body and the brain around pain.

Fortunately, this view is changing due to the International Association of the

---

21 Lorimer Mosley, David Butler, and Timothy Beams, *The Graded Imagery Handbook* (Adelaide, AU: Noigroup Publications, 2019).

Study of Pain (IASP)'s 2020 revision to its definition of pain: "An unpleasant sensory and emotional experience associated with, or resembling that associated with, actual or potential tissue damage."[22]

The IASP further added to the definition that "pain is always a personal experience that is influenced to varying degrees by biological, psychological, and social factors."[23] In other words, the level of pain you experience can be ratcheted up by the following factors.

Biological

- Tissue damage

- Body mechanics (lifting and movement)

- Inflammation

- Poor sleep

- Stress

- Fatigue

- Genetics and body constitution

Psychological

- Thoughts (such as focusing solely on pain)

- Beliefs

- Anger

- Depression

- Boredom

- Trauma

---

22 Angie Drakulich, "Pain Redefined: Inside the IASP's Updated Definition," MedCentral, August 3, 2020, https://www.medcentral.com/pain/pain-redefined-inside-iasp-updated-definition.
23 Drakulich, "Pain Redefined."

Social

- Family's reaction to your situation

- Religious influences

- Personal historical experience with pain

- Treatment by doctors and the health-care industry

- How others view your condition

- Insurance and the disability system

A Snapshot of How Emotions Impact Pain

In 1995, a 29-year-old construction worker jumped on a plank that had a nail protruding from it. When he landed, he was shocked to see that his steel-reinforced boot was impaled by the nail; he had an iron nail penetrating through his boot.

He fell to the ground, writhing in agony. The project manager helped him into his truck and took him to the ER. During the trip to the hospital, every bump on the road increased his misery. At the hospital, he was sedated to remove his boot. When it was removed, it was discovered that the nail had missed the edge of his foot. There was no injury. Despite the absence of tissue damage, though, the agony he experienced was real.[24]

This story demonstrates IASP's expanded definition of pain. Due to the construction worker's thoughts, emotions, context, and perceptions, he experienced pain despite the fact that he hadn't sustained an injury.

---

24   P. Fisher, D. T. Hassan, and N. O'Connor, "Minerva," *British Medical Journal* 310, no. 70 (1995), https://doi.org/10.1136/bmj.310.6971.70.

Living with Chronic Pain Can Scramble Your Brain

Chronic pain is the uninvited visitor who brings nothing but chaos into our world. It's like living with a young child who's learning how to play the violin and has only mastered screeching sounds 24/7. Our neurological warning messengers are busy disrupting our brain and strengthening their presence by recruiting other messengers. These fortified neural networks keep sending their protective danger signals, even though the original injury has long since healed.[25]

The good news is that in the late 1990s, neuroscientists demonstrated that the brain is flexible throughout our lives. In the past, many scientists believed our brain was "hardwired." This means all the neural pathways are set in stone by the time we reach adulthood. The new view holds that we can impact the development of more helpful neural pathways by making use of targeted behaviors.[26] What this means for us as people living with chronic pain is that, using the strategies in this book, we can establish new pathways that will override the errant alert pathways and diminish the false warnings.

As I mentioned in chapter 1, when I heard about the flexible nature of our brain (neuroplasticity), I experimented with challenging my brain with sensory stimulation exercises. Over time, I could tell new pathways were being developed as my pain levels eventually decreased. It was like new neural freeways were constructed, and from that point on, the old neural frontage roads rarely saw a pain message.

This science-based approach is now being used in rehabilitation programs for

---

25   David S. Butler and G. Lorimer Moseley, *Explain Pain*, 2nd ed. (Adelaide, AU: Noigroup Publications, 2013).

26   Moheb Costandi, *Neuroplasticity* (Cambridge, MA: MIT Press, 2016).

brain injuries, post-stroke recovery, and amputees with phantom pain. Many multidisciplinary pain management programs also incorporate neuroplasticity exercises in a treatment protocol called graded motor imagery (GMI). This therapy focuses on sequential exercises of graded intensity that help train our brain to stop creating pain.[27] Another advancement in neuroplasticity occurred in 2023, when a simple-to-use app called TrainPain (www.trainpain.com) hit the market. This affordable app enables the user to perform neuroplasticity training at home.

Case Study: Fibromyalgia

One of my favorite things to do is guest lecturing at colleges. I wear many hats and can lecture on a wide variety of subjects. On one of those occasions, I discussed my personal journey to wellness while explaining how chronic pain impacts family and friends. After my presentation, a male student approached me to discuss his mother Asha's fibromyalgia condition. His mom was a 48-year-old mother of three college-aged students.

Fibromyalgia Syndrome

Fibromyalgia syndrome (FMS) is one of those disorders that creates havoc in a person's life. Not only does it cause muscle pain, tenderness, fatigue, headaches, and sleep disturbances, but it also impacts memory and mood.

This chronic disorder affects up to 6% of the global population, and women are twice as likely to develop it as men are. Currently scientists haven't identified the exact cause of this agonizing condition. Some researchers believe that people with FMS may experience abnormal pain perception processing in

---

27   Ann-Marie D'Arcy-Sharpe, "What Is Graded Motor Imagery and How Can It Help Treat Chronic Pain?" Pathways, December 4, 2019, https://www.pathways.health/what-is-graded-motor-imagery-and-how-can-it/.

their brains. This means their brains misread the SOSs they receive. Regardless of the brain's misinterpretation of the sensations, the pain it emits is real.[28]

Symptoms

- Chronic, widespread body pain

- Moderate to extreme fatigue

- Sleep disturbances

- Sensitivity to touch, light, and sound

- Cognitive difficulties

Risk Factors

- Stress or traumatic events, such as adverse childhood experiences, auto accidents, post-traumatic stress disorder (PTSD), and complex post-traumatic stress disorder (CPTSD)

- Illness

- Repetitive injuries, especially injuries to joints

- Family history

- Obesity

- Underactive thyroid gland

Diagnosis

- Patient history

- Physical exam

- Scans

- Blood work

---

28   Mirjana Dobric, "37 Super Real Fibromyalgia Statistics & Facts for 2023," LoudCloud Health, April 2, 2022, https://loudcloudhealth.com/resources/fibromyalgia-statistics/.

Treatments

- Medications

- Exercising, including muscle strengthening

- Establishing a restful sleep pattern

- Avoiding cold

- Dietary management to avoid processed foods

- Stress management

- Cognitive behavioral therapy to treat underlying related depression[29]

During the early days of the pandemic, I met my chaplaincy clients outdoors to stroll and talk wearing our masks. I called this activity Walk with the Chaplain. It was so successful that I've continued it to this day, though masks are now optional. When I met with Asha, she attended our walk meetings dressed in colorful silk saris. Her gold bangles accentuated the gold thread woven through the silk fabrics. She also wore a bindi, the traditional colored dot worn in the center of the forehead by Hindu women.

She stood at the side of the high school track, her long thick black braid hanging down her back. Her face lit up with a smile as she turned in my direction.

"Namaste." Asha joined her palms in front of her chest.

I bowed back, then we began walking around the perimeter of the school campus to keep her sari from getting dusty from the track.

Asha and her husband had relocated from Mumbai, India, to Northern Cali-

---

29   "All About Fibromyalgia," National Fibromyalgia Association, accessed December 28, 2022, https://www.fmaware.org/fibromyalgia/.

fornia in 2000. Her husband was a successful software engineer, and though Asha had been an English professor in India, she had chosen not to pursue a teaching career in America. In 2005, Asha's widowed mother had joined them in California.

Working with Asha provided an opportunity to understand how culture can impact pain. According to *Hinduism Today*, "Hinduism encourages the acceptance of pain and suffering as part of the consequences of karma." Often, members of this faith tradition aren't forthcoming about their health challenges and prefer to accept them as spiritual growth.[30]

Asha's family was a blend of Eastern and Western culture. They practiced a Hindu vegetarian diet, but they allowed their daughters to wear Western clothes, and they allowed all three kids to be part of American culture outside the family home.

The entire family was concerned about how weary-looking Asha had become. She had growing shadows under her eyes, and her shoulders slumped. Lately, she had become withdrawn and had lost her spark. To support her healing, the family did most of the household duties, leaving her with little to do.

As we strolled down the school sidewalk under the warm afternoon sun, I asked, "What did you think when your son suggested we meet?"

We took several steps before she answered. "He was impressed with your information. He said you were easy to talk to and your pain experience was similar to mine."

"I think it might be." We stopped to let a mother pushing a stroller pass us, and then I asked, "How long ago did you receive your diagnosis?"

---

30 "Educational Insight Part II: A Health-Care Provider's Handbook on Hindu Patients," *Hinduism Today*, January 1, 2013, https://www.hinduismtoday.com/magazine/january-february-march-2013/2013-01-educational-insight-a-health-care-provider-s-handbook-on-hindu-patients/.

She told me that her journey had started around three years before. Her discomfort had first begun in her back and then progressed to her arms and legs. She talked of her struggles to find the right medications and her difficulty even getting out of bed.

"What do you do on your good days?" I asked.

She laughed. "I make up for all the things I cannot do when I'm stuck in bed."

Her behavior is common among people with fluctuating pain. Their good days are chock-full of activities to make up for lost time. This unfortunately means they often pay for it in the following days.

"Would you be willing to restructure your activities to expand your good days and decrease the frequency of your bad days?"

She nodded, and we continued to lap the school as her sari fluttered in the gentle wind. I proceeded to explain that complete bed rest wouldn't heal her condition but would instead make it worse. She needed to add purpose and meaning into her days and participate in life.

On top of telling her to get out of bed, I requested she keep a daily activity journal tracking her discomfort levels so we could see if there was any correlation between her activities and the amount of discomfort she was feeling.

Two weeks later, Asha reported she had held back from overdoing things on her good days and had discovered that, after she paced herself, she didn't have to spend even one day in bed. Her transformation wasn't due to magic; rather, it was being mindful of her activities that reduced her bedridden time.

Asha also made substantial progress in addressing the biological aspect of her condition. She conscientiously performed the strengthening and toning exercises she had received from her physical therapist. She also established a restorative sleeping pattern by turning off her iPad at night and relaxing with a book an hour before bed.

After this substantial progress, it was time to discuss how her diet could improve the way she felt. She was a vegetarian and ate many wonderful anti-inflammatory foods, herbs, and spices, which was beneficial for living with FMS. In our discussion about her food choices, it was revealed that she had a habit of drinking her tea with a lot of sugar and enjoying her mother's savory deep-fried cakes containing bits of cauliflower, onions, and other vegetables as a frequent afternoon snack. After learning about the inflammatory effects of sugar and high-fat food, she decided to omit those things from her diet.

She was doing well with self-care, keeping up her strength-building, and practicing better sleep habits, so we focused on the psychological aspect of her syndrome. She shared that she was being hounded by depression from feeling like FMS controlled her life.

I assured her that it didn't have to stay that way. We could put more structure into her days to support her body's natural healing by using my AIM program. Asha brightened at the thought that she could use the distractions she enjoyed as a powerful tonic for reducing misery.

After working through the steps of the AIM program, Asha signed up with an online tutoring program to help high school students study for the AP English exam. She was able to teach 10 hours a week and never had to cancel a tutoring session due to her FMS.

During our last walk, we discussed the social component of her FMS. Asha said that things had improved with her husband and mother after she explained the physical and emotional aspects of having her condition. They were surprised to hear that structured activities rather than extended bed rest would not only improve her overall strength but also help her moods. For the first time in three years, her husband viewed her as an active participant in their marital relationship. This improved her relations with him, and soon she was able to resume some of the easy household tasks to lighten her aging mother's and children's responsibilities.

Asha also entered into passionate discussions with her mom about their faith. Asha wanted to honor their faith as a moral compass, but to also shed any guilt she experienced from having a health challenge that interfered with her family life. Through these conversations, she was able to find a way to honor her belief by being reminded that her spiritual growth could come through prayer, study, and her tutoring service.

Her story demonstrates that the key to reducing suffering comes from powerful self-care strategies and taking the right healing actions. To be successful with the AIM program requires a shift from thinking that a doctor does all the healing. It means we become proactive and take charge of our health.

To do this requires that we do not put all our hopes into the medical system. The medical system can be part of the solution but not the *total* solution. This isn't an easy quest if we choose to take it on. It's a challenge to adjust our diet and exercise and to practice stress-reduction strategies. These things are even harder when we're hurting.

One thing I know is that the fact that you picked up this book means that you believe change is possible. You've identified that it's time to learn new skills to improve your health and reduce your suffering. In the next chapter, you'll learn how to rewire your brain to change your body's response to the environment. You'll also learn how to flip your negative past into a positive future.

REMEMBER:

- Chronic pain is different than acute pain.

- Chronic pain means your brain is still sending pain messages, even though the body part has healed.

- Emotions, thoughts, feelings, and environment can amplify pain.

- Neuroplasticity provides hope for retraining your brain.

- Addressing physical, psychological, and social aspects can reduce your discomfort.

- We can quickly learn self-management strategies.

CHAPTER 5

Short-Circuit Your Pain

♥

"Every now and then a man's mind is stretched by a new idea or sensation,
and never shrinks back to its original dimensions."
—OLIVER WENDELL HOLMES SR., PHYSICIAN AND POET

Ready to learn how to feel better now, despite your chronic pain? As you learned in chapter 4, the discomfort you're experiencing isn't an indicator of an existing injury that needs to heal. Rather, your two-and-a-half-pound brain is valiantly maintaining its role as protector of your body. It doesn't realize that it's time to stand down after successfully warning you about your original injury. The activities in this chapter will help you retrain your brain to stop sending the old alerts. You'll be able to measure your retraining progress by the fact that you're experiencing less pain.

There are four foundational activities you need to perform in order to do this.

Foundational Activity #1: Set Up a Happy Day

Your outlook can have an enormous impact on how successful you are in improving your health. If you start each day with a negative view about the helpful strategies you're trying to incorporate into your life, you'll negatively influence their outcome.

Here's an example of establishing a positive frame of mind to enhance the positive outcome of the strategies you choose to incorporate into your day.

1. The night before or early in the morning, create a list of the activities you have planned for the day that will improve your comfort. These might include stretching and movement exercises, deep breathing, journaling, or listening to your favorite music.

2. Imagine how each activity will lessen the tension in your muscles, calm your thoughts, and lift your mood.

3. Check off each activity as you complete it. Note any changes in your comfort level.

Performing this simple task will release the feel-good chemical, dopamine, in your brain. Later in this book, you will learn how to access a full range of other biological "happy chemicals."

Foundational Activity #2: The Language of Pain Relief

By the time you've transitioned from an acute state to a chronic state, your brain has been struggling with the physical and emotional aspects of the experience for over three months. The life you once knew has been disrupted, and the simple pleasures and joys in your life have faded away. If you continued seeing doctors during this time, you likely feel like you stepped onto a treadmill of medical appointments where you were reduced to a diagnostic code that doesn't reflect your ongoing suffering between appointments. Whether you continued to go to doctors or not, you may find yourself searching the internet for solutions to end your misery.

Some people spend a lot of time reading through the latest medical findings in the hope they'll discover a cure, only to find themselves depressed when treatment options elude them. Some in a depressed state seek out support and connection through online health support groups. Connecting with others can provide an important social connection. Unfortunately, many of these groups' discussions focus solely on pain levels and frustrations about health care. Just reading other people's negative experiences can stimulate your brain to produce alert signals that something is wrong, which increases emotional and physical distress.[31]

Even more emotional distress can result if we aren't careful about the choice of words we use in our self-talk about our condition.

Here are common words used to describe the feeling of pain:

- Agonizing
- Angry
- Burning
- Crippling
- Excruciating
- Gnawing

- Inflamed
- Raging
- Severe
- Sharp
- Stinging
- Torturous

31   Kristeen Cherney, "Are Sympathy Pains a Real Thing?" Healthline, April 14, 2020, https://www.healthline.com/health/sympathy-pains.

As our brains process these words, our suffering increases due to physiological changes. An example of this is when we suddenly hear a car slam on the brakes. Our heart rate increases, adrenaline surges through our body, and our muscles tense as we anticipate a possible collision.

When we tell ourselves, "I'm in excruciating pain," our muscles tense and our heart rate increases. Our brain is in alert mode and tries to help us cope with the agony we're experiencing. It's difficult to think about treatment options when our brain is shouting.

In my search to overcome the symptoms of my CRPS, I decided to experiment with my self-talk. One morning I was experiencing burning on the left side of my neck all the way down through my left thigh and into my left foot. I sat on my bed thinking it felt like lightning was striking me over and over and fire was raging inside my body.

As I rubbed my neck, wondering how I was ever going to make it through the day, I decided to change how I described the fire in my body. I told myself I felt like embers were smoldering inside of me because my muscles were tight and were pulling at the nerves throughout my body.

By substituting less intense descriptive words like "tight" and "pulling" rather than "lightning striking me" and "raging," I opened my mind to the fact that I could do some things to lessen the intensity. My feelings of frustration about my discomfort disappeared as I alternated heat and ice compresses on my neck and lower back. After that lessened the pain, I used a handheld massage wand to relax my muscles. This turned down the intensity of my complaining body parts. The physical and emotional relief I was able to obtain by changing the way I described my soreness motivated me to suggest this approach to my clients. Each one followed up with me to share that the shift in their self-talk helped prompt them to use comforting techniques instead of sitting in misery.

Here are less intense words you might use and comforting actions that correspond with each.

SENSATION	RELIEF TECHNIQUE
Achy	Heat, pain relief creams
Fatigued	Rest
Sore	TENS unit, capsaicin cream, magnesium baths
Tender	Massage, ice, moist heat (if not contraindicated)
Tight	Stretching, massage, foam roller

Which milder terms would best describe your uncomfortable sensations? As you think of these words, envision ways to reduce the sensations. Changing your self-talk descriptive words can open the door to comforting activities so you can feel better.

Foundational Activity #3: Activating Our Senses

Sensory stimulation refers to the input and sensation received when one or more of our five senses is activated.

Our five senses are:

- Seeing (visual)

- Hearing (auditory)

- Touching (tactile)

- Tasting (gustatory)

- Smelling (olfactory)

Examples of sensory stimulation include when your mood improves upon hearing a favorite golden oldie tune, or when you smell the fragrance of chocolate chip cookies right out of the oven. The senses transport you to a better frame of mind.

Sensory stimulation works because it causes our brain to create new neural connections. Doctors have found this extremely helpful in improving the well-being of people with neurocognitive disorders and pain.[32]

The daily sensory stimulation activities I used when I began my neuroplastic journey included:

1. **Seeing:** Watching bird documentaries.

2. **Hearing:** Listening to songs that held special memories.

3. **Touching:** Wearing soft clothing that soothed the discomfort from my neuropathy.

4. **Tasting:** Sucking on sugar-free mint lozenges.

5. **Smelling:** Wearing aromatherapy lavender oil on my wrists.

A good way to figure out how to do this for yourself is to do a Five Senses Inventory of things you enjoy.

1. **Seeing:** What do you like to look at?

2. **Hearing:** What are the special songs, symphonies, or sounds you enjoy listening to?

---

32 Scott Frothingham, "What Is Sensory Stimulation?" Healthline, September 10, 2020, https://www.healthline.com/health/what-is-sensory-stimulation.

3. **Tasting:** Did you have a favorite gum, hard candy, or lollipop as a child?

4. **Touching:** What feels good on your skin?

5. **Smelling:** Is there a special scent you enjoy?

Foundational Activity #4: Ways to Flex Your Brain

Research shows that the areas of the brain that include focus and attention light up when a person is engaged in a physical or mental exercise. Moving your body through exercise or using your brain as you engage in problem-solving (for example, by completing a crossword puzzle) or creating something (for example, by writing in a journal) strengthens the development of new neural pathways. As these pathways are being developed and strengthened, the other neural pathways that shout "Pain!" weaken.[33] In a later chapter, you'll learn comfortable ways to incorporate movement into your life.

Mental Exercises

- Jigsaw puzzles
- Crossword puzzles
- Computer mind exercises
- Sudoku
- Journaling
- Learning a foreign language

---

33 RIKEN Brain Science Institute, "How Our Brains Keep Us Focused" ScienceDaily, January 22, 2012, www.sciencedaily.com/releases/2012/01/120122104803.htm; Tzu-Wei Lin, Sheng-Feng Tsai, and Yu-Min Kuo, "Physical Exercise Enhances Neuroplasticity and Delays Alzheimer's Disease," *Brain Plasticity* 4, no. 1 (2018): 95–110, https://doi.org/10.3233/BPL-180073.

Case Study: Rheumatoid Arthritis

I received a desperate Instagram message from the adult daughter of a 55-year-old man who'd just received a diagnosis of rheumatoid arthritis in December 2020. The woman's father, Jerry, had undergone a successful bypass surgery a few years before his diagnosis, in 2018.

After the surgery, Jerry quit smoking and adopted a healthy diet and exercise program. Despite all these healthy behaviors, he had a lot of pain in his joints. The doctors diagnosed him with rheumatoid arthritis and told him the pain wasn't from his old college football injuries.

The diagnosis sent him into a depression. He stopped his post-surgery healthy diet and exercise habits and slipped into a doomsday attitude. His daughter reported that this was unlike him. He was a high-powered mortgage broker and a weekend musician.

Rheumatoid Arthritis

There are over 15 distinct types of arthritis, and rheumatoid arthritis (RA) is considered one of the more severe and debilitating forms. In the United States, 1.5 million people cope with this arthritis, which women develop two to three times more frequently than men.[34]

RA's assault on the body is caused by an abnormality in the immune system that turns the body against itself. Antibodies are released that generate chemicals that cause inflammation in the lining of joints by inhibiting the production of the joints' fluid. All joints are at the mercy of RA's attack. Without the benefit of fluid, the joints' cartilage and the connective tissue between the

---

34   Matthew Ezerioha, "Let's Dig Into Everything about RA," Rheumatoid Arthritis Support Network, September 13, 2018, https://www.rheumatoidarthritis.org/ra/.

bones are destroyed, which can result in pain, stiffness, swelling, and damage to the joints and, ultimately, can lead to deformity. A person can also suffer a low-grade fever from the condition. The exact cause of RA is unknown, but it's believed that genetics and environment play big roles.

Symptoms

- Swelling

- Stiffness

- Pain

- Redness

- Other physical symptoms might include fatigue, low fever, loss of appetite, skin rash, muscle aches, and other signs of high levels of inflammation

Risk Factors

- Age (40–60)

- Gender (women are two to three times more likely to get it)

- Family history (if a parent or sibling has RA, one has three to five times higher risk than the general public)

- Smoking

- Obesity

- Hormone changes

Diagnosis

- Patient history
- Physical exam
- Scans
- Blood work

Treatments

- Anti-inflammatory medications

- Surgery as needed to restore joints

- Exercise to strengthen the muscles around the joints

- Stress management

- Sleep pattern restoration

- An anti-inflammatory diet

- Physical therapy

- Cognitive behavioral therapy to treat underlying pain-related depression[35]

After much cajoling by his daughter, Jerry agreed to meet with me over Zoom. I know many people (including me) are challenged by Zoom's technology. Our first meeting would be Jerry's first brush with videoconferencing. As he appeared on screen, I saw he was a very fit giant of a man, probably well over 6'2".

Frustration was on his face, and I read the four-letter words on his lips as he tried to get his microphone unmuted. His smiling daughter's face came into view as she reached across his computer to unmute him. She had the same blond hair and sky-blue eyes as her dad.

Flashing my warmest smile, I said, "Greetings. I'm glad we finally have a chance to meet."

Jerry's daughter thanked me for taking the time to meet with him. As soon as

---

35   Matthew Ezerioha, "RA Treatment: What is the Safest Treatment for Rheumatoid Arthritis?" Rheumatoid Arthritis Support Network, November 2, 2018, https://www.rheumatoidarthritis.org/treatment/.

she saw that he was comfortable with Zoom's technology, she patted his arm, said, "You're all set," and left.

I scanned the room behind him. I noticed all sorts of baseball and football paraphernalia, as well as many photos of him and his daughter mountain climbing. I was looking into the weathered face of a man who obviously enjoyed the outdoors.

"I hear you've recently been told you have RA."

His brow wrinkled. "I couldn't believe it when my doctor told me my knees and swollen hands were the result of having a woman's autoimmune disease." His uttered the word "woman" with disdain.

"You know, many men have RA too, like Sandy Koufax, the famous Dodgers pitcher."

The brow crease lessened.

"How has RA changed your life?"

"I had just lost thirty-five pounds on a heart-healthy diet, and I thought my health was improving, but then I found out I have this lousy condition." He sighed. "I thought that by adopting healthier behaviors, I'd stay healthy."

I could feel and understand his frustration.

"I bet your RA was around long before you adopted your healthier lifestyle."

That caught his attention.

"How long have you had this pain?"

He sat back in his chair, thinking. "Hmm. Ever since my college football days,

I've struggled with my knees and fingers becoming swollen and inflamed. Now it's gotten so bad I've had to cancel playing the keyboard at some of my '70s cover band's weekend gigs." He sighed, clearly frustrated about that.

"My rheumatologist wants to refer me for hand surgery so I can regain mobility in my right hand. I figure, if it won't cure the RA, why bother?" His shoulders slumped.

"It sounds like the surgery would help you continue playing."

"True," he admitted.

"You experienced success when you decided to change to a heart-healthy diet."

"Yeah."

"I have some other things you could try that might make a difference in your quality of life."

Many of the people I work with have multiple health challenges besides pain. If that's your story too, be assured that the tools I'm presenting will help your health across the board.

The first thing I worked with Jerry on was to help him accept the fact that RA isn't a gender-based diagnosis. It did take a bit of convincing, but once he accepted that, his overall mood improved, and he was willing to listen to my advice on how he could lessen his aches and pains. Not long after hearing about the power of using less intense pain words, Jerry told me that when his joints were aching, he now looked at them and said, "It feels like you want to be soothed with warm compresses."

Over the months that we met, he realized that even though surgery couldn't cure his RA, it could improve his life by increasing the flexibility of his fingers so he could continue playing his band's weekend gigs. A month before his scheduled surgery, he incorporated a daily sensory stimulation program into his days.

This is Jerry's sensory stimulation program:

- **Seeing:** Watching reruns of his favorite World Series games.

- **Hearing:** Listening to recordings of his group's best gigs.

- **Tasting:** Chewing Black Jack gum, his favorite childhood gum.

- **Touching:** Wearing his soft velvet robe when he watches his football games.

- **Smelling:** Lighting a pine-scented candle that reminds him of his hikes with his daughter.

Close to the surgery date, I received a note from him thanking me for reminding him to keep a positive outlook about the outcome of the surgery. He had reached out to others who had undergone the same type of surgery, and everyone told him the same thing: "I wish I hadn't delayed in having the surgery." His research led him to tell me, "I just want you to know I'm keeping a positive view about the outcome."

Four months after the surgery, his doctor encouraged him to play his keyboard to strengthen his fingers and increase their flexibility. Jerry was impressed by how much more flexible and comfortable his finger joints were as he played.

During our last meeting, I learned he'd returned to his heart-healthy diet and had also increased his fitness program. He was still implementing his "just in case of a flare-up" activities like memorizing new song lyrics, writing new song arrangements, and researching hiking trails to hike when he felt better. One of the additional activities on this list was connecting with his band members through the magic of Zoom to play a round of song trivia.

The tools I suggested in this chapter are things you, too, can begin incorporating into your life today. Each one puts you in the driver's seat. Not one of them depends on a doctor or a visit to the physical therapist. The next time someone tells you your pain is all in your head, you can respond, "You're right, my brain does generate pain messages, but now I know how I can use neuroplasticity to dampen those messages."

In the next chapter, you'll learn further techniques to reduce negative thoughts and feelings that perpetuate your cycle of pain.

REMEMBER:

- Neuroplasticity exercises will help you.

- Adjust your outlook every morning.

- Use less intense pain words.

- Incorporate sensory stimulation into your day.

- Exercise your mind every day.

CHAPTER 6

Saying Yes to Help Yourself

♥

"You never know how strong you are until being strong is your only choice. "

—ATTRIBUTED TO BOB MARLEY, MUSICIAN

I harbored a persistent hope that the magical combination of medications would be my salvation from the challenges I was facing. But it never happened. Even though I was using my AIM program and the four foundational activities to minimize my suffering, I struggled to get my son off to school, maintain my household, and hold my marriage together.

It took every ounce of my energy to ignore the raging burning in my body while I drove my son to after-school activities and quickly returned home to greet my husband at the end of each day with a home-cooked meal that he'd appreciate after a hard day at work.

One day, leaving the doctor's office and being told to take the same old medications that basically did nothing, I stormed into my car and cried. "Nothing's getting better, and it won't if I keep waiting for them to heal me," I vented to myself and God.

As I waited for some type of answer, I remembered the famous old saying that insanity was continuously doing the same thing and expecting a different outcome. When I remembered that, I couldn't help but think, "Yep, I've been acting insane."

It was time to stop holding on between medical appointments in hopes that they'd make me better. They weren't doing the job, so I was going to have to. I pulled out my textbooks and professional journals to see if I could unearth another hidden gem to help me.

As I reviewed my resources, I recalled a public health professor explaining that doctors were trained to focus on a collection of symptoms, not the total person. If that was true, that meant my doctor's only focus was on pain levels, rather than whether the treatment helped me to fully engage in my life.

I researched to see how things have changed in the past years. What I uncovered was unsettling. A doctor's patient caseload impacts the time that can be spent with each patient. This meant my doctors only had time for a short check-in to update my medical records and order my prescriptions; they didn't have time to strategize on any other part of my health.

Something inside me told me that my health could get better—maybe it couldn't return completely to what it once was, but it could get better. I was willing to do just about anything to improve, but this time I'd expand health research.

On a hunch, I checked out information in the health self-care category. That didn't mean shutting the door completely on the health-care system. They would remain a partner in this quest. Besides, I still needed them to get my prescriptions and lab work so I could monitor my condition with numbers. I also needed my doctor's signature on my biannual long-term disability eligibility forms.

In those days—the late 1980s—it wasn't as easy to supplement my knowledge about pain management as it is today. The public didn't have access to the internet then. I visited medical school libraries and spent a fortune copying professional journal articles that could give me insight on how to improve my life. When I finally had access to the internet, I scoured medical and physical therapy sites for useful information. Since YouTube wasn't launched until 2005, it would be years before I'd have access to the amazing array of useful scientific presentations that can now be found on that platform.

When I created my personal self-care program, I set a schedule to review my materials at the Mill Valley Depot Café and Bookstore. This got me out of the house and gave me a sense of purpose. During those review sessions, I had my TENS unit set at high intensity and my left hand wrapped in an ACE bandage to protect it from changes in the temperature. I tried to ignore the discomfort of sitting for an extended period of time.

Because I had a computer, books, and journals spread out in front of me, people got the impression I was an author. Their curiosity would get the better of them, so I was often asked about the subject of my book. I was happy to share my latest ideas about overcoming chronic health issues. This always generated interesting conversations. I became privy to stories about bad backs, bad knees, autoimmune illnesses, and mental health challenges.

One woman was especially intrigued by the information. She had ongoing problems with her back. She was excited when I gave her an outline of my self-care program, including the three action plan–creation questions, which we'll discuss more later in this chapter. She promised to look it over. Imagine my surprise when she sat down at my table weeks later and handed me notes about how she had successfully used my program and asked me to include her story when I finally did author a book.

Here's her plan for improving her chronic bad back.

- What did the doctor say about her condition?

Her doctor diagnosed a slight bulging disc and age-related degenerative discs. Surgery wasn't recommended. She was instructed to give up playing tennis, her favorite sport. To treat her discomfort, she was advised to take Tylenol or Advil for flare-ups and to learn to live with the aches of an aging body.

- How could she improve her health?

She researched pain management options and learned that she was a suitable candidate to receive an epidural steroid injection (ESI) into the space around her spinal nerves. This injection numbed her nerves and provided relief. She also researched body mechanics. She learned to refrain from lifting heavy objects. Since she works from home, she invested in a special office chair that provides lower back support.

- What areas of her life did she want to improve?

She missed playing tennis, which had given her a sense of accomplishment and provided her with a social outlet. Seeking to replicate this experience, she researched types of exercises that wouldn't aggravate her back. She discovered a strengthening and toning program that loosened up her back so she could participate in her favorite weekly spinning classes.

She was able to construct an improvement program by using the three basic questions as a guide. She applied her simple plan and found more happiness in her life and a reduction in her pain. She also said that she planned to use this successful approach for any future health issues.

Hearing her success gave me the courage to continue on my quest for myself. If my research was helping someone else, I felt confident that I could improve my own life quality even more than I already had.

I reviewed my status again. I had been told that the nerve damage from my neurological condition was permanent. My dominant left hand, with its permanently swollen joints, was useless. It turned ice cold regardless of the weather. Whenever storms rolled in, my hand turned bright red and swelled like the Pillsbury Doughboy's hands, and the whole left side of my body also felt like it was on fire 24/7.

If the physical pain wasn't enough, the surgery I underwent to cure my condition cut and sealed a portion of my sympathetic nerve chain in my left side collarbone area. This left me with something called Horner's syndrome. This condition manifests as a permanent drooping of my left cheek and upper eyelid. Additionally, the pupil in my left eye remains permanently constricted, which I discreetly conceal with glasses. The surgery also permanently altered my voice. Despite these challenges, I've learned to adapt and persevere.

This condition is so unusual that many doctors have only seen it in a text-book. That makes me a novelty when I walk into their exam room. When my surgeon noticed it at my postoperative checkup, he casually mentioned that I could undergo plastic surgery to fix it. After I reviewed the literature and learned that any type of surgery could further spread my burning symptoms, I knew I'd have to live with the changes in my appearance.

The dissection of my sympathetic nerve chain also prevents me from perspiring on the left side of my face, so the other side overcompensates. I have to constantly mop the moisture on my right side, regardless of the weather. Living through the hot flashes of menopause was crazy. I was dry as a desert on the left side, and the right side was a constant monsoon.

I'd been promised that the surgery would cure my pain, and I had trusted the surgeon with my life and genuinely believed he was going to improve my health. Instead, he turned me into one of Pablo Picasso's avant-garde paintings of distorted faces. I could hardly dare look into a mirror. The horror of the situation weighed heavy on my shoulders.

Trying to shake that off, I sought out additional health-care information beyond what I was getting from my health-care providers. I learned that when doctors are trained in medical schools, they receive less than five hours of pain education. These courses concentrate on surgical interventions and drugs for pain management, but they fail to address the psychological and sociological aspects of chronic pain.[36]

Because my doctors lacked the knowledge I needed, I read everything I could and then created my own plan of action to feel better by answering the following questions:

- Where am I now with my health status?

In other words, what are my doctors saying about my condition?

- How can I improve my health status?

In other words, what kind of information about my condition and treatments can I find on the internet, YouTube, and in libraries?

If the idea of doing research is scary because you don't have a science background, don't worry. Many medical schools, health-care systems, and disease research foundations continuously post updated information online geared toward us laypeople. Not only will you not need a medical dictionary to understand their articles, but they also provide scientific links to back up their facts.

---

36   Erika Halonen, "The Problem of Pain Education," Aivo, August 16, 2022, https://aivohealth.com/blog/the-problem-of-pain-education; Judy Watt-Watson and Beth B. Hogans, "Current Status of Pain Education and Implementation Challenges," International Association for the Study of Pain, July 9, 2021, https://www.iasp-pain.org/resources/fact-sheets/current-status-of-pain-education-and-implementation-challenges/.

- What areas of my life do I want to improve?

In other words, what changes can I make that will help me physically and/or emotionally?

Answering these questions gave me a map to guide me toward improving my health. I know it will do the same for you, just as it has for many of my clients.

Case Study: Central Post-Stroke Pain

I moved into my friendly new neighborhood in Dublin, California, a region 36 miles east of the San Francisco Bay, in 2018. Every day, I noticed an 85-year-old woman, Lori, walking her two Welsh Corgis. This senior woman wore her hair in an elegant gray bun and had a lean and fit body envied by neighbors half her age. We often waved to each other, and we developed a personal connection in August 2019 when I officiated her neighbor's funeral at the local heritage cemetery.

Standing with her son on the pathway in front of gravestones from the 1880s, she greeted me. "I didn't know you were an interfaith minister," she said. "I thought you were an artist."

I smiled at the other neighbors as they passed by. "I consider myself primarily a spiritual person who embraces life."

After that day, when she spied me sitting on my porch, she stopped by for pleasant extended chats or sought healing prayers for her friends.

In April 2020, she showed up at my door, her usual tidy gray bun lopsided, with loose strands hanging down her face.

I opened my door to her and asked, "What's wrong?"

"It's my son, Dale. He's not doing too well."

Dale was a burly man with graying hair. He was a 52-year-old widower. At the funeral, he had worn his Harley-Davidson jacket even though it was 82 degrees beneath the Japanese elm trees. All his mom's senior neighbors doted on him because they could depend on him to fix their cars, their garbage disposals, and their cable TV problems.

Lori told me that her boy had had a stroke over Thanksgiving, which had left him with a drop foot (a foot that drags due to nerve damage) and difficulty with his speech, along with an overall weakened body. Not long after the stroke, he had moved into his mom's house to recover since his house had multiple stories.

Dale had done physical, occupational, and speech therapy and was improving. Research suggests that patients make the most significant recovery progress in the first three to six months of stroke rehabilitation.[37] But at the six-month mark, in April, during the early days of the pandemic, he had developed central post-stroke pain.

Central Post-Stroke Pain

Central post-stroke pain is a chronic neurological pain syndrome resulting from damage to the central nervous system.

The disease affects up to 8% of stroke patients and can occur weeks to months after the event.[38]

---

37 Preeti Raghavan, "Stroke Recovery Timeline," Johns Hopkins Medicine, accessed March 13, 2024, https://www.hopkinsmedicine.org/health/conditions-and-diseases/stroke/stroke-recovery-timeline.
38 "Central Poststroke Pain," American Academy of Physical Medicine and Rehabilitation, accessed March 13, 2024, https://www.aapmr.org/about-physiatry/conditions-treatments/pain-neuromuscular-medicine-rehabilitation/central-poststroke-pain.

Symptoms

- Feelings of aching, burning, pins and needles, numbness, or stabbing affecting the face, arms, legs, trunk, or even an entire half of the body

- Constant pain

- Intermittent stabbing sensation

- Worsens over time

- Can be aggravated by touch, temperature changes, movement, and emotions

Risk Factors

- Stroke

- Multiple sclerosis

- Tumors

- Epilepsy

- Brain or spinal trauma

- Parkinson's disease

Diagnosis

- Musculoskeletal and neurological physical examination

- Brain imaging

Treatments

- Pain medications offer little relief

- Tricyclic antidepressants

- Anticonvulsants

- Lowering stress levels

- Mindfulness-based cognitive behavioral therapy (MCBT) for depression and anxiety[39]

In early March, Dale felt pins and needles digging into his skin. He also experienced burning, tingling, and pain that felt like a dentist was using a sharp instrument to explore an exposed nerve in a tooth, except he was feeling it in the back of his neck and not in his mouth.

He was frustrated and angry because the doctor wanted him to treat these sensations with an antidepressant or an anticonvulsive medication rather than with opioids.

Lori had been his cheerleader during his grueling early rehabilitation work and had helped him celebrate every improvement, but now his condition was quickly declining. She asked if I could talk to him about his pain in person since his speech was too difficult to understand over the phone.

There had been a regional shelter-in-place order in effect since the end of March, so I met people in their driveways rather than entering their homes. I'd arrive on my bike dressed casually, wearing my mask. My choice of clothes was to protect the privacy of the people who I was helping. I wore shorts or jeans to camouflage the fact that, while sitting in driveways, I might be discussing end-of-life health directives due to a private terminal cancer diagnosis, or arranging a memorial, or helping someone decide to make the gut-wrenching decision to place their spouse who was suffering from Alzheimer's into a memory care facility.

It was a chilly April day when I rode up to meet Dale. He sat on a folding

---

39   "Central Pain Syndrome," National Institute of Neurological Disorders and Stroke, accessed February 16, 2024, https://www.ninds.nih.gov/health-information/disorders/central-pain-syndrome.

chair, decked out in his leather jacket and a mask. Leaves were just appearing on the trees along the street, and his mom's garden was full of tulips and daffodils. He chuckled as he noticed the stuffed cat attached to my knapsack on the back rack of my bike. When I had embarked on my pandemic undercover chaplain role, I had added the cat prop so that people would have a reason to smile under their masks.

I pulled off my bike helmet and tried to puff up my flattened curls as I sat across from him on the lawn. Lori's dogs, Abbott and Costello, barked when they heard my voice.

"How're you doing, Dale?"

Although his speech was halting, I could understand his description of his central post-stroke pain symptoms and his disgust about the medications he was being offered.

I reached into my knapsack and pulled out a folded-up diagram of a human body I'd filled out years ago to show my doctor the areas where I was experiencing unpleasant neurological sensations. I held it up, and his eyes opened wide as he studied all the red, orange, and yellow spots representing different intensities of burning pain.

"It's unbelievable to see that another person's patterns are similar to mine. How's that possible?" he said.

"I'm not a physiology teacher who can explain why the distribution of our neurological sensations is similar, but I can be a member of the team helping get you closer to your recovery goals."

He glanced at his Harley-Davidson sitting idle on his mom's driveway and sighed.

"I hear you've been working hard using special exercises to recover your speech and you also got fitted for a brace to help you walk with your drop foot."

A deep frown edged onto his face. "I was making really good progress until the burning started."

"Let's talk about how you can continue making progress."

The first thing I talked about was how some classes of antidepressants and anti-convulsants are amazingly effective in calming down unpleasant nerve sensations and are often prescribed for many different types of nerve syndromes.

"I thought the only thing that could help was opiates," Dale muttered.

"Well, so far, you're seeing improvements with your speech and physical therapy, and I bet you can do even better by adding a self-care program into your existing rehab program. The steps of this type of program will help guide you to gather up more information about your challenges and help you discover solutions so you can overcome them."

I explained the questions in the self-care program I had designed. Dale already had up-to-date information about what his doctors were saying about his condition, so I assigned the next question: "How can I improve my health status?" Researching his syndrome would educate him about the use of helpful medications and therapies.

"The libraries are closed right now, so that's impossible." He groaned.

"It's all at your fingertips on the computer."

He confessed that he was a book and magazine type of guy (he especially loved classic motorsport magazines) and didn't enjoy sitting in front of a screen typing all day.

"It will only take a few strokes to type 'central post-stroke pain' and then hit enter. I'm sure you'll find a list of patient education information on the subject that you can either read on the screen or print."

He agreed to give it a try.

We met the first week of May, sitting in the shade of his mom's porch where the geraniums and azaleas were in full bloom. Dale unfolded our lightweight chairs so we could sit across from each other and then, without thinking, he picked up notes he had dropped.

"You're feeling better," I said, stating the obvious.

"I'm taking Neurontin, an anticonvulsant, and it's making everything less intense, especially the feeling like an exposed tooth nerve."

"That's great to hear."

He nodded. "Did my homework," he blurted out. "Learned it's possible to change neural pathways, which means my speech will continue to improve. Not only that, but I also learned my vintage Z/28 Camaro can be adapted so I can drive it with my drop foot."

He overflowed with excitement about what he'd learned as he breathlessly shared that he was fascinated by neural pathways because they reminded him of the electric schematics he referred to in his auto work. This research led him to a free brain training app online, Luminosity (www.lumosity.com/en/), which helps you increase the flexibility of your brain simply by playing games using a phone's touch screen. Dale signed up, and now a new game appears on his phone every day.

"I sit on my front porch and people think I'm texting, but I'm really strengthening my brain."

When we'd last met, Dale said that his physical therapist wanted him to begin walking in the neighborhood with a walker with wheels to strengthen his body and improve his coordination and balance. When I observed that he wasn't doing this, he said, "I'm not using a walker like my mom's friends use."

A neighbor walked by and greeted Dale with, "It's wonderful to see you looking so well."

After exchanging some small talk, we got back to business.

"How about pushing around Abbott and Costello's dog stroller to help you balance?"

Now, that may sound like a big ask of a guy, but our neighborhood is full of offbeat people who stretch the limits of convention like I do by having a unicorn in my yard and riding around with a stuffed cat on my bike.

"Fine. At least it's not an old geezer's walker with wheels."

That day we reviewed the final question of the self-care program: "What areas of my life do I want to improve?"

Dale pointed to his bike. "The answer is sitting right there. Someday I want to be strong enough that I can feel the wind raging against my body again as I roar through the back roads on my bike."

"Walking and listening to your favorite music to get your strength and balance back will help you get there."

"I'm a Bob Seger guy, so I'll listen to *Night Moves*."

Dale and his dog stroller became a common sight in the neighborhood, and our meetings drifted to a monthly ongoing check-in on the phone. Dale often said that following the program I suggested helped him feel in control and taught him that there is a whole wide world of things to research beyond Harleys. Every now and then, he texts me when he finds new brain training programs that are offering discounts so I can let others take advantage of these resources.

I developed my self-care approach due to my frustrations with being stuck. If you're at that point, it's time to answer the three basic questions and start moving forward in reclaiming control of your own health. Again, these questions are:

1. Where am I now with my health status?

2. How can I improve my health status?

3. What areas of my life do I want to improve?

So far, we've covered how the mind can increase suffering. In the next chapter, you'll learn how to use the same simple mind-body techniques that helped me overcome negative thoughts and the trauma I experienced from the facial nerve damage caused by my surgery.

REMEMBER:

- Self-care means you're confidently taking charge of your health needs to live a healthier lifestyle.

- By answering the three simple questions, you'll have your personalized map to guide you to improving your health.

- If you surf the internet, you can find updated information about your health challenge.

- You can make a positive change in your life.

CHAPTER 7

Shift Your Thinking

♥

"We become what we think about."

—EARL NIGHTINGALE, SPEAKER AND AUTHOR

Fueled by the success I found in my self-care program, I continued to gather up the latest scientific information to help solve my health problems. In between poring over journals at medical libraries, I prowled the growing self-help aisles in bookstores.

My search didn't let me down. I hit gold when I discovered the book *Seeing with the Mind's Eye: The History, Techniques, and Uses of Visualization* by Dr. Michael Samuels, a leading pioneer in holistic healing, and his wife, Nancy Samuels. It taught me that creativity, visualization, and guided imagery can be potent techniques for healing.[40]

The book inspired me to buy a guided imagery cassette tape (I didn't own a

---

40   Michael Samuels, *Seeing with The Mind's Eye: The History, Techniques and Uses of Visualization* (New York: Random House, 1975).

CD player). The tape combined bilateral music (more on that in chapter 15) with a pleasant New Zealand–accented narrator. He guided me to close my eyes and imagine colors and comforting sensations. I laid with a pillow under my knees to relieve the pressure on my lower back.

My African grey parrot kept me company by perching on my knee as I listened to the soothing sounds. My muscles relaxed, and the intensity of my burning subsided. I listened to the tape every afternoon for years. When I learned that the tape was no longer being sold, I made duplicates in case it broke.

Years later, I was excited to learn that Dr. Samuels would be lecturing at a local event. Immediately, I signed up and took a front-row seat, soaking in one moving story after another about how creative arts and guided imagery aided his patients who faced life-threatening illnesses.

Dr. Samuels took the audience through a live demo of a guided imagery exercise that lessened my pain. After the demo, a brochure and application for a new interfaith chaplaincy seminary were handed out. The curriculum covered interfaith spiritual care using many of the creative arts and healing traditions discussed in the Samuelses' book.

Chaplaincy, as I discovered to my delight, isn't an exclusive club—it's a broad, interfaith practice embracing all faith traditions, including my Jewish faith. But chaplains don't just provide services to those dealing with illness or trauma; they also lead ceremonies for weddings, rites of passage, and funerals; organize interfaith services; and drive educational programs.

The moment I heard about this inclusive approach, I was super excited. My background in public health and counseling was perfect for such a role. Plus, the best bonus of all, chaplains could work part time.

I enrolled on the spot, already daydreaming about doing the work that would be so fulfilling it might boost my efforts in my own healing journey of reducing my pain.

At this juncture, my marriage, already strained due to my CRPS, reached its breaking point. My Austrian husband harbored a lifelong dream of returning to Europe and traversing the globe. I, however, didn't share this vision. We parted ways on amicable terms, and I channeled my focus into a new journey—pouring 100% of my efforts into my studies at the Chaplaincy Institute.

Three weeks later, I arrived for my first day of class prepared for the long days of learning. I was armed with my ever-faithful TENS unit and a handcrafted lace gauntlet adorned with pearls and attitude to camouflage my protective sling on my left hand. Seated regally atop an inflatable exercise ball like a queen on her throne, I continuously adjusted my posture for comfort. Hours clicked quickly by as I soaked up the information I felt lucky to be learning. My classmates thanked me for giving them a unique perspective on what it was like to live with a chronic condition. They said it would help them understand their patients' challenges better.

Ours was the inaugural class. We were on the ground floor of a program that would expand over the years. We studied the roots of world religions to give us the knowledge to interact on an interfaith basis. This background empowered us to navigate the spiritual care of our diverse community members, regardless of their faith traditions. I developed expertise on how best to make use of spiritual music, song, dance, and creative arts to assist in healing.

Only a month after being proudly ordained as both a chaplain and an interfaith minister, I was recruited as an on-call police chaplain. My job was to provide spiritual and emotional support to traumatized children and women whose lives had been touched by tragedies like serious accidents, violent acts, or family members struggling with mental health issues. The night before my first ride-along with an officer, the anticipation of having the privilege of serving the public was so intense that sleep decided to take an impromptu vacation.

It's amazing how affixing my shiny chaplain badge on my starched white regulation police shirt and then donning my black jacket with "Police Chaplain" in huge letters across the back magically made my own discomfort diminish, as if it had hailed a cab and left the scene. My noble mission was clear: to bring comfort to lessen the trauma the victims experienced. I relished that role, and soon those ride-alongs became the highlight of my weeks.

So, there I was, suited up in my uniform, riding along with officers and ready to offer solace and be the calm amidst chaos. I always had a pocket full of finger puppets, my secret tool for winning children's trust to be able to guide them into a relaxed and emotionally secure space. My most successful cases were when the kids taught their parents the breathing relaxation tools I'd taught them. Seeing those little faces light up with a glimmer of hope, witnessing their worries melt away, made it all worthwhile. Those moments were shots of espresso to the soul.

But there were other aspects of the job where it was impossible to make a difference. Sometimes things were heartbreaking. Life as a police chaplain was like being on a roller coaster that filled my heart with reverence for the human spirit. It also gave my life a whole new meaning.

At the same time, as I dove into the world of police chaplaincy, the American Pain Society, a group of renowned scientists, clinicians, and other professionals, stated that pain should be considered the "fifth vital sign" and that screening for pain was as important as screening for the other four vital signs—body temperature, blood pressure, pulse (heart rate), and breathing rate (respiratory rate).[41]

Some states decided to shake things up and passed Intractable Pain Treatment Acts giving doctors the green light to use opioids for chronic pain patients like yours truly. Meanwhile, in a parallel universe called "Pharmaland," pharmaceutical companies were on a marketing rampage, downplaying the risk of opioid addiction while emphasizing their benefits as a safe, effective option for pain relief. The result? A sudden surge in the number of opioid prescriptions being scribbled on doctors' pads.

Dr. Redhead digested the information presented by the drug company sales rep and then contacted me with an offer of the pain medications Norco and fentanyl, the Holy Grail for effective relief. On that day I thought, "This is monumental. I'll finally be pain-free."

I understood that along with my two different antidepressants I'd been taking for years for nerve pain, I'd initially be prescribed a low dosage of fentanyl patches that could be bumped up over time. Accepting this prescription meant I had to return to the clinic every month since the prescription didn't come with refills.

At first, every time I left the visit with script in hand, I believed I was on my way to achieving a pain-free existence. I was hoping this was so when, after a few weeks, I noticed that my spasms felt less intense. Unfortunately, with the lessening of my muscles complaining, my burning shouted as loud as ever. My doctor countered this by upping my dosage, and before long, I wore two large patches, all the while popping Norco, my "breakthrough pain" medication, every four to six hours.

As I neared the six-month mark, the dark truth set in that, in my case, the

---

41   David W. Baker, "The Joint Commission's Pain Standards: Origins and Evolution," The Joint Commission, May 5, 2017, https://www.jointcommission.org/-/media/tjc/documents/resources/pain-management/pain_std_history_web_version_05122017pdf.

medication wasn't going to get me out of pain. In fact, the dual opioids barely scratched the surface. Not only that, but when my fentanyl dosage was increased, I suddenly had rivers of sweat pouring down me as if I were a basketball player in the fourth quarter of a hotly contested game.

The first time I noticed this alarming side effect was on a police chaplain call-out. To my horror, I felt my uniform shirt clinging to my back. I ducked into a bathroom and stood in front of the electric hand dryer to dry myself to appear calm and collected. If the clinging shirt wasn't bad enough, picture me interacting with traumatized people while mopping the perspiration off my face.

My hyperhidrosis (excessive sweating) caused Dr. Redhead to advise me to change my patches every 48 hours rather than the customary 72 hours because my flood of perspiration was affecting the dosage level. He also suggested I get Botox injections, which, besides being used for cosmetic purposes, also treat hyperhidrosis. Those injections come with a caveat about possible nerve damage, so that wasn't happening. My body didn't need further damage.

When I declined the injections, Dr. Redhead wrote me a prescription for a blood pressure medication that also treated hyperhidrosis. That turned into a no go because it made me dizzy. I ended up coping with my perspiration predicament by gathering up a collection of vintage designer handkerchiefs and using them to mop my brow. I was creating a new kind of fashion state-ment with my growing collection of lace gauntlet arm sling covers and my Christian Dior hankies.

During one of my monthly prescription pickups, the doctor asked how my chaplaincy work was going. When I referred to a current traumatic case that made the headlines, he said he knew that my heart and head were all into my work. He asked if I thought the stress was impacting my pain.

The truth was that I was hanging on by my fingertips. Every call-out came at a huge physical cost. After each event, I was bedridden for days until I peeled myself off my bed for the next call-out.

My driving force was that the police officers depended on me—both for the expansion of the interfaith police chaplain program and for my distinctive approach to soothing traumatized children.

I was making a difference by helping people during the most traumatic days of their lives, yet it was coming at a great cost to my physical well-being. I reluctantly put my uniform aside and pivoted to the less stressful world of community chaplaincy work by teaching other health sufferers to implement self-care strategies to improve their lives. Although the choice was incredibly hard to make, it has felt right, and I don't regret it because it provided me with the opportunity to create a practice based on my training in health science, counseling, and spirituality. This combination of training has proved invaluable in meeting the needs of my clients, who are seeking to improve their quality of life despite their chronic illness diagnoses.

In the middle of all this change, I got married to my "mind-blowing sex" husband, Len. This required a shift to a different insurance carrier and connected me with Dr. Wise-and-Caring. The new carrier required me to be assessed by a multidisciplinary medical team in order to be eligible to stay on my opioid regime.

It turned out they couldn't deny the impact my self-care practice had on my condition. They waived the requirement to attend pain management classes. I knew, and so did the doctors, that my self-care tools were helping, and fentanyl wasn't eliminating my burning sensations. I continued to research in order to add additional strategies.

By early 2010, a national storm was brewing over opioids. While some cases require management with opioids, I suspected they were being over-prescribed. I knew the truth about these potent medications. They weren't harmless and weren't the complete wonder drug that the advertisers hawked, and they created physical dependency.[42] The consequences of being under their influence would become evident whenever a patient's medication supply was disrupted due to their pharmacy's lack of stock. A sudden stoppage of their opioid prescription found them enduring excruciating withdrawal symptoms, which often triggered desperate behavior for patients to get their hands on the drugs.

One tragic story after another appeared in the news, covering the untimely deaths of people who had been prescribed fentanyl, Norco, or OxyContin for pain issues resulting from bad backs, auto accidents, or work site or high school sports injuries. Long-term usage of these drugs led to tolerance. Due to this, sometimes higher doses were necessary to obtain the original amount of relief. The singers Prince and Tom Petty are examples of people who over-dosed in pursuit of finding relief from their painful hip conditions. Still other overdose deaths occurred when desperate chronic pain patients sought relief in street drugs that were lethal counterfeit versions of opioids.

It's a heartbreaking reality that, as I write these words in 2023, some patients find themselves compelled to withdraw from opioids due to evolving regional regulations. These regulations were created in response to the national opioid crisis and are impacting the availability of medically necessary prescriptions.[43] Patients with opioid prescriptions have to search far and wide to find a pharmacy that has their specific drug in stock.

Online support groups are popping up where patients share information about drugstores that have adequate inventory. They also share names of clinics that still manage pain with opioids. Many health clinics are instructing

---

42   Emily Campbell, "OxyContin Created the Opioid Crisis, but Stigma and Prohibition Have Fueled It," The Conversation, August 31, 2021, https://theconversation.com/oxycontin-created-the-opioid-crisis-but-stigma-and-prohibition-have-fueled-it-167100.

43   "Guidelines for Prescribing Controlled Substances for Pain," Medical Board of California, July 2023, https:/mbc.ca.gov/Download/Publications/pain-guidelines.pdf.

their doctors to stop prescribing opioids. This shift in medical practice places these patients at risk. Suddenly discontinuing or rapidly decreasing opioid doses, commonly referred to as "tapering off," leads to severe withdrawal symptoms. The abrupt halt of opioid therapy without adequate patient support and alternative pain management strategies jeopardizes the patient's health and safety.[44]

Drawing from my personal journey of successfully tapering off these drugs, which I delved into in chapter 1, I firmly support the implementation of a national medically supervised and gradual tapering program. Such an approach aims to mitigate the profound physical and psychological toll that accompanies the withdrawal process.[45]

The decision regarding usage of opioids should be based on individualized patient care. The physician needs the power to make a clinical judgment, and the patient needs to be informed on proper use and overdose risk. Additionally, their family/caregivers should be educated about the use of Narcan, a medication used to reduce the effects of opioids in the event of an overdose.

Even though relying on opioids didn't help me reclaim an active life, there are reports that use of these medications can be helpful for some chronic pain patients.[46] Since my nine-year detour being on opioids overshadowed my self-care practices, I became even more committed to learning more about the secrets of the brain's connection with the body.

44   Nita Ghei, "The Other Opioid Crisis: How False Narratives Are Hurting Patients," *Discourse Magazine*, July 18, 2022, https://www.discoursemagazine.com/culture-society/2022/07/18how-false-narratives-about-opioids-are-hurting-patients/.

45   Beatrice Aswati, "How Pain Led to an Opioid Epidemic: Learning from the Past to Better Treat Pain in the Future," Science in the News, January 7, 2021, https://sitn.hms.harvard.edu/flash/2021/how-pain-led-to-an-opioid-epidemic-learning-from-the-past-to-better-treat-pain-in-the-future/.

46   Erica Jacques, "Types of Opioids Used for Chronic Pain Relief," Verywell Health, last modified May 23, 2022. http://www.verywellhealth.com/types-of-opioids-chronic-pain-medications-2564496.

I was an explorer hunting for the hidden path to health that I knew in my heart of hearts had to be there. As I continued my hunt, I found scientific journal articles discussing how the brain churns out chemicals. These chemicals stimulate emotions that range from happiness and joy to sadness or even terror. Each one of these emotions changes our blood pressure, respiration, and immune response and can diminish or intensify the body's sensations.[47]

What does the brain's effect on our emotions and body systems have to do with our pain? That's a question I became obsessed with answering. I had a theory: our lives would be more comfortable if our brains generated more positive emotions, like they do when we win a jackpot.

As I read articles about positive emotions, I knew mine were few and far between. I decided to generate more positive emotions and see how that affected my pain levels. To do that, I went on a hunt to tame my negative thoughts and emotions. That's when I found mindfulness-based cognitive behavioral therapy (MCBT).

Before we get going on that, I want to give you a little spoiler: MCBT did lessen my pain and physical symptoms. Not only that, but my loved ones experienced relief too as my suffering lessened. Bonus point.

MCBT: How to Talk to Your Brain

MCBT was developed in the early 2000s by a team of psychologists who combined mindfulness-based stress reduction (M) with cognitive behavioral therapy (CBT).[48] This team of psychologists believed combining both of

47 Jeffery Berk, "Do Feelings Influence Physical Health?" Psychology Today, November 9, 2021, https://www.psychologytoday.com/us/blog/emotions-and-your-health/202111/do-feelings-influence-physical-health.
48 "Mindfulness-Based Cognitive Therapy to Prevent Depression," University of Oxford Research, accessed March 12, 2024, https://www.ox.ac.uk/research/research-impact/mindfulness-based-cognitive-therapy-prevent-depression.

those modalities would result in a potent weapon that would calm down the fight-or-flight reaction in the brain. They found that this technique was helpful for people suffering from depression, anxiety, phobias, and pain.

This approach doesn't heal injuries or illnesses, but it equips individuals with the ability to train their nervous system to be less reactive. Using this training keeps our reactions calmer when we experience uncomfortable remarks made by our bosses, are cut off in traffic, or even get frustrated with glitches in software programs.

To do this technique, you'll start by becoming mindful of what is happening in your body and thoughts (you'll learn how to do this later in this chapter). Then you'll use CBT methods to help you identify and change negative thought patterns and behaviors that can amplify your brain's interpretation of pain signals.

When we use this training, the brain slows down knee-jerk reactions to give us time to accurately assess the threat of danger and choose the most appropriate action. When we have more control, we are reshaping our brain's response patterns and can then navigate life's challenges with more grace, poise, and presence.[49]

All this science brings great news to people on opiates. MCBT has been found to help patients become less reliant on medications. Many doctors are now suggesting that pain patients go to psychologists who specialize in MCBT. However, it's disheartening to note that some medical insurance companies don't cover the cost.

Despite this financial challenge, numerous fundamental MCBT techniques are readily available on platforms like YouTube, allowing you to practice them

---

49 Jae-A Lim et al., "Cognitive-Behavioral Therapy for Patients with Chronic Pain," *Medicine* 97, no. 23 (June 2018): e10867, https://doi.org/10.1097/MD.0000000000010867.

conveniently in the comfort of your home for free. These skills will empower you to pinpoint your triggers and gain a deeper understanding of how to effectively respond.[50] These resources allow you to take proactive steps to reclaim control over your reactions. This in turn helps manage the anxiety, depression, and hopelessness that's often experienced by people living with chronic pain.

Self-Care Tool #1: Five-Minute Diaphragm Breathing

Diaphragm breathing relaxes your nervous system by encouraging the complete exchange of oxygen. When we breathe deeper, more oxygen reaches our bloodstream, and more carbon dioxide leaves the system. This reduces the tension and stress that tightens neck and back muscles. It also lowers blood pressure and increases energy. Finally, it calms down the fight-or-flight response and triggers the body to rest and digest. This is referred to as down-regulating your nervous system. To have a long-term effect, diaphragm breathing should be practiced every day.

Set a five-minute timer and make yourself comfortable, either sitting or lying down.

1. Place your hands on your stomach.

2. Take a deep breath to extend your stomach and expand your rib cage.

3. As you slowly release your breath, imagine your neck and back muscles releasing tension.

---

50 Wen Chen, "Mindfulness Meditation Reduces Pain, Bypasses Opioid Receptors," *NCCIH Research* (blog), National Center for Complementary and Integrative Health, March 16, 2016, https:// www.nccih.nih.gov/research/blog/mindfulness-meditation-reduces-pain-bypasses-opioid-receptors.

Repeat this exercise for at least five minutes to give your muscles time to relax. If you find five minutes is too difficult, then start with two minutes and work up to five.

Consider using this simple type of breathing whenever you find yourself in a stressful situation.

Self-Care Tool #2: Body Scan for Knowledge

In this exercise you'll be scanning through your body for information. You're listening to parts of your body. Is it tight? Hurting? Needing attention? Not feeling well? Or is it doing well? The scan gives you information on where tension is being held in your body. Plus, it gives you a way to slow down your heart rate, lower blood pressure, and decrease the release of stress hormones. This lessens anxiety.

1. Lie on your back with your legs extended and your arms at your sides, palms facing up.

2. Using gentle breathing, start at your scalp and move your attention down one body part at a time to release any tension. Keep this up until you reach your toes.

3. Ask yourself:

    a. Are my muscles tight?

    b. Is any tightness generating discomfort?

    c. Is my pain shouting or whispering?

    d. Does adopting deep breathing lessen the sensations?

e. How am I feeling after releasing the tension?

Self-Care Tool #3: Cultivate a Moment-to-Moment Awareness

When we become aware of what is going on around us, we are cultivating mindful awareness. By doing this, we're changing our brain patterns from the familiar to the unfamiliar. When we enter into the land of the unknown in this way, two things happen. First, the unknown distracts the brain from sending out pain messages, so we experience less pain. Second, it trains our brain to handle stress better and recover faster.[51]

To train the brain, choose a daily task that doesn't take a lot of thought. Pick something like brushing your teeth or washing the dishes.

Change how you do the task. For example, use your nondominant hand to brush your teeth or to hold the sponge as you wash the dishes.

As you perform your task, you will most likely notice how difficult it is to do simple movements. Your focus will be consumed with trying to do the task, which will slow down the brain's pain messages. Each time you can achieve a less painful state, you are resetting your pain alarm system, which is training your brain to keep you in less pain.

Self-Care Tool #4: Deep Dive into CBT Exercises

Living with any type of health challenge is exhausting, and it's difficult to be positive all the time. But the problem is, if we allow our pain to put us in a bad mood, it causes chemical reactions that create even more tension, and that equals more pain. These thoughts also decrease our immunity. So,

---

51 Jeremy Smith et al., "The State of Mindfulness Science," *Greater Good Magazine*, December 5, 2017, https://greatergood.berkeley.edu/article/item/the_state_of_mindfulness_science.

stopping them in their tracks is an excellent idea and something we can do by challenging them.

Here are the nine most common groups our negative thoughts can fall into:

1. **Catastrophizing:** Thinking a situation is worse than it actually is and believing it will have the worst possible outcome. Example: "The sky is falling!"

2. **Discounting the positive:** Overlooking the positive and concentrating on the negative. Example: "I only had two areas move into the healthy range on my blood panel study; five of them stayed in the unhealthy range."

3. **All-or-nothing thinking:** Thinking in extremes and believing that either you must be perfect or you're a failure, or everything is all good or all terrible. "I'll always be in pain, and I'll never be healthy again."

4. **Tunnel vision:** Focusing only on negative aspects of a situation, person, or event. Example: "I'm still in too much pain to sit through an entire concert."

5. **Prematurely negative labeling:** Assessing that a situation or a person is bad without knowing more about it or them. Example: "I didn't like how that doctor didn't smile in his picture. I'm not going to like him."

6. **Responding to a situation based on emotions instead of facts:** Emotions can whisper that you're worthless, useless, hopeless, shameful, guilty, clueless, and unlovable. By checking out the situation based on facts rather than through the lens of your emotions, you'll have a clearer view of how to assess the situation. Example: "No one is going to want to maintain a friendship with a person

who's often not feeling well."

7. **Magnifying a situation:** Assuming a situation is worse than it really is. Example: "I'm going to feel awful forever, and I'm sure I'll spread this lousy condition to my children."

8. **Mind reading:** Presuming you know what others are thinking without having any evidence or interactions with them. A common result of this is to believe that others are always criticizing or judging you. Example: "I don't want to go to the neighborhood party. None of them want to talk to me since I'm so often in pain. They don't want to be reminded that someday they could have their lives upended like I did."

9. **Personalizing:** Thinking you are responsible for situations or events that are beyond your control. Example: "It's my fault I have this condition. If I hadn't spent summers digging ditches when I was young, I wouldn't be in pain now."

Looking through the list, we can see all sorts of ways we bring dark clouds to our thinking, whether by distorting the truth, throwing a wet blanket on things, or becoming too critical. After learning how that way of thinking could increase my pain, I put my thinking process under a microscope.

I immediately understood that I entertained those pain-increasing thoughts from sunrise to sunset. I'd start the morning predicting that I wasn't going to feel well enough to get anything done and then criticize myself for how I approached family situations. I'd round off the day by declaring that my facial nerve damage would never get better.

This observation shocked me. I had never considered myself a negative person, but as I listened to the endless rattle of my thoughts, it was obvious that I was swimming in a toxic bath of my own creation.

I shook my head, thinking about the grip those nasty thoughts had on me. Quickly, I decided to go after the thinking error causing me the most harm: mind reading. If a client showed up angry or sad, it had to be *my* fault. They must think I wasn't good enough to help them, and maybe they had only chosen to work with me because I was more affordable than the bigwigs at a glittering prestigious hospital or highly recommended health agency.

In truth, I had no idea why my clients were angry or sad, and I needed to stop making everything about me because their moods most often had nothing to do with me. That settled, I thought I was good to go, but the very afternoon I came to that conclusion, a client slammed his car door as he hustled over to me on the track.

I heard a brusque "Hello."

I looked over at my client's red face. I told myself, "Bonnie, this isn't about you. Something happened right before our appointment that got him frustrated."

Sure enough, after I greeted him, he told me that when he was ready to leave for our appointment, his car wouldn't start. He used his portable charger, but his car wouldn't take a charge. He called AAA road service and paid through the nose for a battery change in his driveway.

Yes, there were more times clients came in with heightened emotions, and there were more times I talked myself out of taking it personally. In fact, now, when someone appears grumpy, I automatically assume it has nothing to do with me. Another point for me!

Countering my negative thoughts worked so well that I decided to go after my huge anxiety about public speaking. Remember, the left side of my face was droopy and my voice sounds raspy. I was afraid that people would make negative comments about my appearance and my voice.

I reminded myself, "People have come to listen to your lecture looking for hope. When they find out you were hit by a drunk driver and learn about the recovery you fought for, they'll see you as inspiration."

Slowly, as I extinguished my negative thinking, my moods improved and I returned to being the upbeat person I had been before the pain.

Self-Care Tool # 5: Putting All the Steps Together

Keeping track of our moods and our pain levels can help us identify patterns and can aid in our quest to reduce our suffering.

Use a daily calendar to monitor pain, thoughts, and emotions throughout each day. If you note what you are thinking and feeling every four hours, you will see a pattern emerge over time. I was surprised to discover that I struggled in the late afternoons. I learned to schedule activities that would challenge my mind and distract me from the midafternoon cascading negative thoughts.

Pinpointing the times when negative thoughts are likely to erupt and then planning powerful ways to distract is not only fun, but it works. Perhaps you feel bad at the beginning of the day and then feel an improvement by lunchtime. If so, ask yourself what triggers the negative thoughts in the morning.

Talk back to those negative thoughts and figure out a way to start each morning in a better mood. Maybe put on your favorite type of music as you go about your morning routine. Or maybe you need time on your porch with your coffee and space to listen to the birds sing. Whatever will put you in a good mood, make sure to sneak it into your morning.

If afternoons put you in such a grouchy mood that you want to get away from yourself, then ask yourself, "What would make afternoons more fun?" Would it be whipping up a snack? Doing a mini exercise routine to get the blood flowing? Or maybe taking a catnap so you feel refreshed to finish the rest of the day? If evening is the time everything goes to pot, go to bed and sleep away the angst. Maybe you are challenged with sleep; then you might want to soak in a warm tub or open up an irresistible book.

> *"The mind is everything. What you think you become."*
> —UNKNOWN

Case Study: Phantom Limb Pain

A worried police officer contacted me about his dad, who was an elderly retired Air Force major. I learned that his dad had had his left leg amputated due to bone cancer. He was fitted with a high-tech prosthesis that helped him walk with a natural gait, but unfortunately, three months later, he started experiencing phantom limb pain (PLP).

This aggravating condition was driving him nuts and making it impossible for him to coach his grandson's basketball team or host his famous weekend barbecue parties. He spent an increasing amount of time sitting on the sofa drinking beer to "help" his opioids, but they weren't working. He asked for a stronger dose, but instead of getting the prescription, he was referred to a CBT-based rehabilitation program offered by the Department of Veterans Affairs (VA). In the first session, he stormed out, claiming the program was too "fluffy" and "full of hippie nonsense."

Phantom Limb Pain

An amputee often spends months to years adjusting to their missing limb. Some of them have brain-scrambling pain messages telling them their missing limb is hurting. The suffering is real and feels like "tingling, throbbing, sharp, pins/needles…severity varies."[52]

This is a double whammy to the patient since the limb is gone but it's hurting like it's still there. Scientists believe PLP is the result of jumbled signals between the spinal cord and the brain. The brain misreads incoming signals from the body and deciphers them as being generated by a nonexistent limb.

Symptoms

Sensations in the missing limb that might be described as…

- Aching

- Burning

- Vise-like

- Pins and needles

- Throbbing

Risk Factors

- Peripheral nerve trauma

- Spinal cord trauma

- Brain changes

- Psychogenic factors such as depression, anxiety, and increased stress

Diagnosis

- Physical exam

- Scans

---

52   Aaron A. Hanyu-Deutmeyer, Marco Cascella, and Matthew Varacallo, "Phantom Limb Pain," StatPearls, August 4, 2023, https://www.ncbi.nlm.nih.gov/books/NBK448188.

Treatments

- NSAIDs and prescription pain relievers

- Muscle relaxers

- Spinal cord stimulation and TENS

- Mirror therapy

- Complementary therapies: acupuncture, biofeedback, massage, Mindfulness-Based Cognitive Behavioral Therapy [53]

The major was a big man in his late 80s with a full head of white hair and thick wrinkles that showed a lifetime of determination and will. On our first videoconference meeting, he started out by saying, "My son told me you probably weren't into that new age bunk I heard about at the VA. That's the *only* reason I agreed to meet with you. If you dish that out, I'm gone. I'm not happy you're a woman, but I'll overlook that fact for my son's sake."

I leaned back in my chair and took in his gruffness. "Well, I'm glad you're here. I hope you find it helpful since everything I'm going to suggest is based on hard science."

His eyes flickered.

"If you'd like, I can send you links so you can read articles that include brain scan photos that document the regions of the brain that light up and change when you use these strategies."

He chewed on my words, then said, "Okay, I'll read them." His steely gray eyes, which looked like the ocean on an overcast day, peered into me. "You can't imagine how strange it is to feel burning in an ankle that isn't there."

---

53   "Phantom Limb Pain," Cleveland Clinic, accessed January 27, 2023, https://my.clevelandclinic. org/health/diseases/12092-phantom-limb-pain.

He shook his head. "Sometimes it even feels like pins and needles are sticking into the bottom of my nonexistent foot."

"That must be disconcerting."

The hard wrinkle in his forehead lessened. "It is."

"I know you love to coach your grandson's basketball team."

"My grandson's a great forward. He's 5' 11" and is only in eighth grade."

"Wow. That's impressive."

He nodded.

"Should we talk about some of the things that can get you up off the sofa and back to coaching?"

"Okay. But I'm not interested in doing yoga. The VA gave me a list of suggested mindfulness activities. I couldn't believe yoga was on the list. That's against my church's beliefs."

Yoga originated as an ancient Hindu spiritual practice for balancing the mind, body, and spirit. Studies have shown that weekly yoga classes can not only improve mobility for people suffering from lower back pain, arthritis, and other conditions, but can also improve their mood and psychosocial well-being.[54] Because of yoga's origin, some people feel that practicing this mindfulness activity puts them in conflict with their faith tradition.

"The important thing is that you get to choose activities that you'll be comfortable doing."

---

54 "Yoga for Pain Relief," Harvard Health Publishing, April 29, 2015, https://www.health.harvard.edu/alternative-and-integrative-health/yoga-for-pain-relief.

So, we dove in. The major told me more about his situation, and I gave him options for practicing mindfulness and CBT. He immediately chose to focus on his negative thoughts. As we explored his thinking through his health journey, he suddenly declared, "Wow, I'm drowning in a tide of negative thoughts."

"Want to stop them?" I looked at him head-on.

He stared down at his pencil. "Sure."

"This week, create a list of all the negative thoughts you can think of, like the thought that you'll never be back on the basketball court, or the thought that you'll never be able to host parties again. Then I want you to think of ways to counter all those thoughts." I also told him to spend some time doing activities with his nondominant hand to cultivate moment-to-moment awareness.

"Will do."

Over the weeks that followed, he taped his list of negative thoughts to his bathroom mirror and got to work countering them. During our next meeting, he bragged that he had applied military precision and created a two-in-one exercise. He talked back to each negative thought as he brushed his teeth with his nondominant hand. He had effectively combined the mindful immersion exercise with the identifying negative thoughts exercise.

After he implemented those, he became hooked on finding ways to incorporate mindfulness habits and CBT tools into his life. His goal was to deconstruct the assignments to make them his own. For example, he made a battle plan to attack his pain by entering into his deep breathing exercises with visualizations that focused solely on his victorious flights in the Korean War. During a battle in "MiG Alley," he engaged in air-to-air combat with Soviet MiG-15 jet fighters flown by enemy combatants. He recalled the heart-pumping experience moment by moment as he valiantly fought and protected our country.

When he relived those moments, all his PLP sensations evaporated. He described this unique personalized approach to me as he waved his vintage Korean War victory log with stamps representing the five enemy aircraft he had downed in my direction.

"My days in the Air Force made sense to me. I responded to situations based on facts, and I didn't assume a situation was the worst. Even during the hardest times in the war, when us guys in the air were gutting it out, our buddies were being hit hard on Pork Chop Hill, and so I did what needed to be done to protect them."

The profound sacrifice encapsulated in his words stirred a deep well of gratitude within me. His time in the Air Force, a period defined by pragmatism, resilience, and unyielding bravery, was a testament to his indomitable spirit. His unwavering belief in the necessity of his squadron's actions, despite the gut-wrenching realities they faced in the skies, served as a stark reminder of the strength inherent in our servicepeople.

I was witnessing that same indomitable spirit showing up again as he fought for his health for his and his family's sake. But he did hate the paperwork of documenting his thoughts, feelings, and PLP sensations.

I challenged him to try documenting for a week and, if he found it didn't help, I promised I'd never bug him about it again.

To shut me up, he gave it a go.

A week later, he announced that he noticed that the tingling and itchiness of his missing foot started up at 3 p.m. every day. That used to be his coaching time.

"How do you spend your time now?"

He looked sheepishly at me. "I stare at the clock and feel bad."

The major discovered that his PLP symptoms soared when he was bored or missing his old life.

To counter this, he stopped drinking beer and limited his time sitting on the sofa. Instead, he researched his great-uncle's participation in the WWI American Expeditionary Forces.

His relative had arrived in Europe in 1917 to help Britain and France at a pivotal time. The major looked forward to sharing the information with his son and grandson and considered authoring a book based on the WWI diaries that the Library of Congress has placed online. That lessened his PLP symptoms and gave him a sense of purpose. He even sent me links to stories about military chaplains.

The major saw the MCBT tools as a secret weapon against his personal war. He returned to the VA, famous for their innovative methods of helping veterans with limb loss. While on his mission to discover ways to fight his condition, he discovered the ultimate war weapon: the mirror box.

The mirror box is a box with a mirror on one side. The box is placed alongside the remaining limb and, as the patient looks into the mirror, the reflection of the limb makes it appear as though the limb is still there. This tricks the brain into believing the amputated limb is intact and healthy. When the brain registers the limb, it stops sending pain signals.

"It's amazing!" the major reported after he received his mirror box. "I wiggle my right foot and I see both feet wiggling. I use the diaphragm breathing while I concentrate on my brain paving healthy neural pathways over the pesky PLP neural pathways that generate the phantom pain every day."

MCBT and the mirror box got the major back on the court with his grandson and his winning team.

Although every case story I present involves a different health challenge, the tools I describe work across the board, regardless of the disease or condition. If you have any doubt that you will be able to improve your health by using MCBT, visualize yourself experiencing a flare-up and then visualize the relief you'll feel simply by lying down and breathing deeply for five minutes, thinking calm, positive thoughts. That feeling of relief is yours for the taking.

In the next chapter, you'll learn an additional way to face down a flare-up by hacking your body's feel-good chemicals.

REMEMBER:

- MCBT creates positive changes in your brain through neuroplasticity.

- Your thoughts and emotions impact your body.

- There is a variety of mindfulness exercises that you can choose from.

- You will decrease your pain by talking back to negative thoughts.

- Incorporating pain-relieving exercises into your life can be unique and individualized.

CHAPTER 8

You Can Create
Your Happy Tools

♥

"Be happy for this moment. This moment is your life."
—ATTRIBUTED TO OMAR KHAYYAM, MATHEMATICIAN, POET, AND PHILOSOPHER

Let me share a secret with you that I rarely ever talk about. When the pain coping strategies started making my life significantly better, hope surfaced, and my days improved. But as each day slipped away, the night battle against insomnia began, whether I wanted to engage or not. Insomnia was a fierce opponent who won most scrimmages and showed up almost every single night. Persistent little scamp.

Despite the fact that he'd been winning for years, I was hell-bent on discovering how I could defeat him and dream my nights away. My new tactical plan was simple and focused—get as much sleep as possible, even if it was as elusive as gripping onto sand. Instead of being swept away into dreamland, I'd lie awake in the darkness, staring at the ceiling twisting and turning from the cacophony of spasms and burning sensations. Come sunrise, despite how exhausted and horrible I felt, I willed myself to get up and make sure my son made it to school. In a later chapter, I'll share with you how I finally won my battle to get shut-eye every night.

Before I got anywhere near victory, though, sleep bankruptcy dogged me. Even though I had no reserves, I did everything I could to show up for my son so he'd feel loved and supported. That meant attending his basketball games, sitting on the lowest level of the bleachers in case I needed to exit quickly.

What frequently struck me was the glaring contrast between me and the other parents, who sat high up in the bleachers with smiles and carefree chatter. As I watched them, I always found myself wondering if they could even imagine what it was like to feel a searing fire course through their necks, shoulders, and lower backs. I assumed most of them never worried about disappointing their children because they had to retreat to their cars to avoid becoming a public spectacle from the pain ripping through their bodies.

I was obsessed with the chasm that had emerged between my world and the healthy world. The sense of living in another universe of suffering increased with the constant demands to attend the corporate dinners of my then-husband. My role was to present myself as a vivacious spouse who could comfortably converse with the other executives and their partners.

I almost choked on the pressure to hide my pain during those events so as not to negatively impact my husband's career. I needed to reflect that his home life was stable and that he had the support he needed to continue his climb up the corporate ladder.

Part of the stress was not only to appear pain-free but to figure out what to wear that would hide a TENS unit. It had to be a two-piece outfit in order to give me the ability to clip the unit's control box on my waistband. I needed ready access to the unit's dials. Throughout each evening, I would constantly turn up the electrical stimulation volume to drown out my body's complaints. With my short stature, it was hard finding dressy two-piece outfits that would meet my requirements and not require costly alterations. The challenges weren't limited to just my wardrobe, either. The daily effort to keep my attitude and mindset strong weighed heavily on those days when I was too worn out and everything became too much.

Borrowing a baseball analogy, my health, full of random bolts of fire that drained my energy, wasn't hitting it out of the park. So instead of batting a thousand, it was more like I was batting 500.

Picture my daily energy as 500 points. Points were allotted to each task based on the energy it required. Despite my best efforts to conserve my points, I often found myself going into the negative column by evening. Sometimes I was in the negative before the day had even begun.

This game of limited energy versus daily tasks played out like this.

Shop at a Grocery Store

- Drive to the store, ignoring the pain and paying attention to traffic = 50 points of coping energy loss

- Ask for help to lift a quart of milk into the grocery cart = 10 points of coping energy loss

- Reach for a produce bag = 3 points of coping energy loss for each reach, 5 reaches total (15 total points)

- Open the bag with one hand to bag produce = 20 points of coping energy loss

- Load the food on the grocery belt = 200 points of coping energy loss

- Drive back home, ignoring the pain and paying attention to traffic = 50 points of coping energy loss

- Take bags in and put food away = 500 points of coping energy loss
- **Loss of Energy** = 845 points (345-point energy deficit)
- **Result:** Exhausted and unable to move off the bed

Shop at a Mall

- Drive to the mall = 50 points of coping energy loss
- Circle the parking lot to find a spot close to the entrance to my destination = 100 points of coping energy loss
- Walk into the mall = 250 points of coping energy loss
- Study the store map for my department = 20 points of coping energy loss
- Browse the clothes racks and select items to try on = 200 points of coping energy loss
- Try on clothes = 500 points of coping energy loss
- Pay for items and exchange pleasantries with cashier = 300 points of coping energy loss
- Drive home = 50 points of coping energy loss
- **Loss of energy** = 1470 points (970-point energy deficit)
- **Result:** Back to bed

Activity with My Son

- Pick out a movie we both want to see = 25 points of coping energy loss
- Drive to theater = 50 points of coping energy loss
- Purchase tickets and snacks = 100 points of coping energy loss
- Sit in pain and watch a movie for two hours = 500 points of coping

energy loss

- Drive home = 50 points of coping energy loss

- **Loss of energy** = 725 points (225-point energy deficit)

- **Result:** Back to bed

Most days, even though relaxation exercises and talking back to my annoying negative thoughts helped ease my back spasms, thanks to my burning and the overall pain, my coping energy was in the negative column.

I needed more help to tame my response to my body's inferno. I kept asking myself, "What else can I try that's based on science?"

One morning, mulling over this, I drove back from the morning carpool flinching in pain. I'd always held off taking my morning dose of muscle relaxant when I was doing the driving, worried about the possible side effects. After dropping the kids off at their school, I flicked on the radio to distract myself from the increasing discomfort. I caught an interview with Norman Cousins, the author of *Anatomy of an Illness: As Perceived by the Patient*.

When he was editor-in-chief of the *Saturday Review*, Cousins had been hospitalized for a painful tissue disease that surfaced after he completed an intense international assignment. While in the hospital, he experienced incessant noise and being constantly poked, woken up for tests, and fed almost inedible food. The environment aggravated him so much that he told his doctor his hospital stay was worsening his condition. He negotiated a move to a hotel with periodic returns for lab work.[55]

Holed up in his hotel room, Cousins dove into studying the intricate world of brain chemistry and learned that, just like an uninvited party crasher, stress

---

55 Norman Cousins, *Anatomy of an Illness: As Perceived by a Patient* (New York: Norton & Company, 1979).

could come in and wreak havoc on the body. This got him thinking: if mental distress had the power to harm the body, could a happier mindset help it?

Cousins paid closer attention to his moods and realized that the happiest he ever felt was when he was laughing so hard that his sides split. A joke book? Nah, that just wasn't going to make the grade. So he decided to take his laughter therapy up a notch. It was time to transform his hotel room into the venue for an epic comedy film festival of one.

Picture this: it's the 1960s, and Cousins is huddled in front of a projector (because the concept of Netflix is still far in the future). He has reels of *Candid Camera* lined up, surrounding him. *Candid Camera* is a show notorious for catching people's befuddled reactions to outrageous practical jokes, and the sight of people being unwittingly pranked had Cousins erupting in belly laughs. His discomfort took a back seat. With his mood hitching a ride on this laughter express, he ventured further down the comedy lane.

Now, the Marx Brothers were the legends of laughter, so naturally, the Marx Brothers comedies of the 1930s were his next stop. With each comic antic, he laughed so hard he could swear his laughter lines had laughter lines. But here's the kicker: these knee-slappers didn't just have him in stitches; they also lured him into such a state of relaxation that his fear of never being able to accept another writing assignment slipped away. Talk about comedy paying dividends.

His film festivals helped him because he wasn't just indulging in a comedy marathon; he was also flexing his gray cells, which improved his neuropathways. His health was restored, and he credited laughter as his magical healing elixir. This experience launched him to author a book about his humor experiment that attracted international attention.

He didn't invent the concept that emotions can influence health, but his work received positive worldwide acclaim. Scientists saw credibility in his idea, and in 1978, he was recruited as an adjunct professor in the psychiatry and biobehavioral sciences department at UCLA.[56]

Lucky for me, I had a perfect opportunity to set up my own epic comedy film festival inspired by Cousins's so I could see if it would work for me, too. My husband and I had an upcoming trip to Maui. Traveling was hard on my body and often caused increased flare-ups. To counter this grueling pattern, before we left, I bought stand-up comedy videos to play.

As soon as we arrived at our condo, my husband took off snorkeling. I plopped onto the couch and watched the funniest of the videos I had brought to calm my complaining body. My husband came back from the beach shaking off sand, a bit pink, his stress lines fading. I greeted him with a grin, feeling a lot better than I had when we had first arrived. From that point on, I packed a film festival every time I traveled.

Finding so much relief from using comedy when my body felt it had been rolled over by a steamroller, I wondered if I could play with the concept of a "runner's high" some of my friends talked about. Was there a way I could have that kind of high without vigorous exercise? Once I got back from my restorative trip to Maui, I headed to the medical library to research if that was possible.

Research indicates that an intense sense of happiness and pleasure can result from an extended period of exercise.[57] It turns out that we can also experience "a runner's high" from swimming, water aerobics, cycling, and other aerobic exercises. The idea of water aerobics caught my eye because I swam competitively in high school. With my muscle weakness from my CRPS, swimming laps didn't feel doable. Instead, I joined a water exercise class that was held in

---

56 Shari Roan, "The Positive Influence of Norman Cousins," *Los Angeles Times*, December 6, 1990, https://www.latimes.com/archives/la-xpm-1990-12-06-vw-8306-story.html.

57 Kelly McGonigal, "Why Does Running Give You a High? A Look at the Science," TED Ideas, April 28, 2022, http://ideas.ted.com/why-does-running-give-you-a-high-heres-the-science/.

a heated indoor pool. Later in the chapter, you'll learn about the therapeutic value of water.

The first day I walked into the pool building smelling the chlorine, hearing the familiar pool sounds, and feeling the humidity, a sense of nostalgia hit me. I hustled to my class, wanting to get into the water that had been my friend for so many years. But as I made my way there, I also felt a tinge of apprehension, wondering if this was a smart idea. The last thing I wanted to do was to bring on a flare-up.

I quickly slipped into the water and started chatting with other class members, forgetting my doubts. Halfway into the class, doing non-weight-bearing exercises, I was thrilled to realize that the buoyancy of the water was making me feel steadier on my feet than I had felt in years. My classmates claimed that the same thing was happening to them too. All of us laughed good-naturedly at ourselves as we attempted the various exercises. By the end of the class, instead of being in serious pain and drained, I glowed with an "exercise high."

My overall pain was reduced as a result of the happy film festivals and water exercise program. But I still had a serious lingering issue that I wanted gone— the sensation like a blowtorch fire that was burning the left side of my body. That intense pain kept me scavenging for what else I could do. I kept reading the research and noticed frequent articles about how much pet companionship created a positive effect for people living with chronic pain.

As a chaplain and health educator, I witnessed firsthand how pets enriched the lives of my clients. I love animals and wanted that experience too, but at that time, I was allergic to cats and dogs.

The solution to my pet dilemma was solved on a beautiful fall day. The air was crisp, and red and orange leaves were floating to the ground. A friend and I stopped by a new pet store to pick up supplies for her dog.

Standing on a perch by the cash register was a green-and-lilac parrot next to a sign that read, "My name is Sammy." I've been fascinated by birds ever since I was a five-year-old and met Polly, my neighbor's talkative yellow-and-green Amazon parrot.

The bird greeted me. "Hello. How ya doing?"

Laughing, I said, "I'm doing well. Aren't you a gorgeous bird?"

"Want him?" the teenager managing the cash register asked.

The pet store was actively searching for the perfect home for the much-loved Sammy, who had a birth defect in one of his wings that made him unable to fly. Unfortunately, his owner's asthmatic condition had deteriorated to the point where she couldn't care for the little bird's lively needs.

I stared at the colorful bird, knowing I wanted him but also wondering if I could handle the awesome responsibility of owning an exotic pet. Luckily, desire outweighed caution, and I heard myself saying, "Yes!"

That afternoon, I welcomed the little green-and-lilac guy into my home and heart. The next day, he launched into antics, mimicking his past asthmatic owner's coughing and wheezing, making me amused at his skill and sad for the previous owner. I loved Sammy so much that I transformed my garage into a vibrant air quality–controlled aviary and welcomed five more special-needs parrots into my life. They form a cheerful and bustling flock, making my garage into a lively place. As I write this, they are thriving and cherished and make me smile.

My parrots lift my spirits and amaze me with their sensitivity to my moods. When I share stories about their antics, people often share their own stories of how their rabbits, horses, or ferrets provide them with joy, expanding my former limited belief that only cats and dogs can be good human companions.

Pet therapy led me to explore other strategies over the years, including music, gardening, and the expressive arts, to see how they could make me and my clients feel better. "Expressive arts" is a term used to refer to the creative activities a person engages in to improve their physical, mental, and emotional well-being. It includes a variety of artistic modalities such as visual arts, dance, music, theater, storytelling, and poetry.

My chaplaincy training taught me how to use expressive arts in the spiritual context, but I had yet to incorporate them to diminish my pain until my stepdaughter Leia introduced me to Bluetooth. I learned that, by using special earbuds, I could listen to music from my phone or tablet without being attached with wired earphones. Since I was already dealing with wearing two long TENS unit wires down my back, it was great to be free of using wired earphones.

The earbuds helped me enjoy streaming music without the cumbersome wires while taking my walks, grocery shopping, and waiting for service in long lines. Favorite golden oldies from the 1970s became my go-to soundtrack. I found out how powerful music is when I was stuck in a slow-moving line at my bank. The Spencer Davis Group's song "Gimme Some Lovin'" serenaded me as I covertly tapped my foot.

When I was newly married to Len, we lost our lawn to a drought. I hated seeing the dirt. The ground in our front yard mirrored what my life had become since my pain had appeared—barren. I wandered around my house feeling stripped of vitality for years, but now, since I had implemented a growing number of helpful strategies, I was on the mend. Maybe I could heal my front yard too.

I decided to visit the Ruth Bancroft Garden in Walnut Creek for inspiration. It's renowned for displaying extraordinary succulents and drought-tolerant plants that are accentuated by artistic sculptures that complement the natural beauty of the landscape. The day after I visited, I looked out onto my desolate front yard and couldn't help but think about transforming my yard into that type of wonderland. I began making plans to create a vibrant garden full of colorful art projects.

As I strolled the perimeter of my sloping yard, the weeds scratched my ankles, and I pictured scraping away weeds and thorns to create a new yard with thriving plants and artistic garden accents. Just thinking about all the different species of birds I could attract with the types of plants I used brought a broad grin to my face.

Deep purple salvias were going to be a main attraction because they're a magnet for hummingbirds. I'd also add manzanita shrubs to provide shelter for ground-dwelling mourning doves. Wanting to hide the chain-link fence on the border of our property, I decided that climbing jasmine, with its tiny white flowers providing a sweet fragrance to the air, would be the perfect camouflage. Best of all, I'd include a small teak bench so I could sit and be surrounded by the best nature could offer while I greeted my neighbors.

To bring my vision to life, I turned to good old YouTube to discover how to cultivate happy plants. The wealth of information I gathered helped me create a plant schematic that had my yard divided into sections, including a meandering hedge of salvias and a slightly elevated area for a Japanese maple so it could tower above the yard. The easy part was going to be lining up the jasmine next to the chain-link fence.

Plans in hand, I headed to Home Depot. While hunting for my plants, I saw a board covered with landscape architects' business cards. One's bold print bragged about having the lowest prices in California.

The tight garden budget I had could barely cover hiring my neighbor's high school son to dig holes for me, but I decided to check the landscape architect out. The business owner turned out to be not only a landscape architect but also an auto mechanic and stand-up comedian. He agreed to review my plans for an incredibly low fee, and he also offered to come meet me at a nearby wholesale nursery, where his business license allowed him to help me purchase my plants at a steep discount. (You'll hear more about him in a later chapter.)

The money I saved on the plants made a difference. I was now able to pay for my young hole digger to spread weed-blocking fabric and mulch to keep the weeds down after Len enthusiastically volunteered to put in a low-cost do-it-yourself drip irrigation system he'd learned about on YouTube.

With my trusty Bluetooth earbuds in, I danced to Playing for Change's collection of up-tempo rock music as I floated around the yard directing the planting of all the plants I had fantasized about. Gradually, my barren yard morphed into an oasis of vibrant flowers that attracted hummingbirds and admiring glances from neighbors.

As my yard transformed, I couldn't wait to do the art accents! Accents are the secret weapon to infuse a garden with personality. My goal was to make my captivating garden pop with quirkiness. I wanted my garden to be a place where I loved spending time and felt just like myself.

To add a whimsical touch, my young helper placed heart-shaped stepping stones to form a curving pathway. Then I gathered up vintage teapots and colanders I'd been collecting for the last two decades. With just a touch of soil, we turned them into one-of-a-kind pots filled with white, orange, and lavender miniature roses. To my delight, word quickly spread about my fantasy garden, and people of all ages came to check it out.

Next, I hit the thrift shops for animal figurines, and I assembled a veritable zoo of figures ranging in size from a one-foot monkey to a three-foot elephant. I lovingly rejuvenated each one with easy-to-use outdoor acrylic paints (no prep needed). Freshly restored in coats of bright blues, oranges, and purples, these colorful animals proudly claimed their place in the yard. I used the remaining paint to cover the stones with inspirational words and phrases like "hope," "you rock," and "blessings."

Suddenly, King Julien from *Madagascar* and Queen Elsa from *Frozen* appeared alongside the thrift store animals because the neighborhood kids had decided to donate their favorite toys to be on display. The most dramatic donation was a five-foot-tall vintage carousel horse that I converted into a magnificent blue-and-white unicorn. Standing next to the unicorn became the kids' favorite spot to pose for pictures.

One late afternoon, as the sun cast its last rays over my garden, a young mom approached me as her kids played hide-and-seek between the plants and decorations. After some small talk, she asked if I'd mind her photographing the garden to practice her photography skills. I was thrilled and soon grew to appreciate her eye. I admired what she saw in my mystical haven. It didn't take long for her photography career to take off, and she was able to make a good living with it. She gifted me some of her early photos, and they still hang in my office.

My initial plan for playing gardener had been to get rid of a patch of unsightly weeds while distracting myself from my health challenges. At no time had I envisioned that I'd be creating an opportunity to build a flourishing social life. My neighbors began visiting my enchanting garden and asking me for gardening advice. Apparently, my unique approach to gardening inspired them to remove their water-thirsty lawns, try their own low-maintenance drought-resistant gardens, and adorn their yards with statues and other repurposed objects. Every time another front yard was converted from a plain patch of browning lawn to a lush perennial garden, Mother Nature smiled.

Landscaping a front yard is a major physical and financial undertaking, but you don't have to take on this type of mammoth project to reap the benefits of being out in nature and enjoying vegetation. Later in the chapter, you'll learn less taxing, lower-cost ways to enjoy plants, sunshine, and fresh air.

♥

"Never, ever underestimate the importance of having fun."
—RANDY PAUSCH, PROFESSOR AND MOTIVATIONAL SPEAKER

Life Enhancement Program: Personalize Your Self-Care Strategies

Above, you read about how I created a life enhancement program that was tailored to what makes me happy. Now it's your turn to be happier. This program is about seeing what's possible for you, going after more of the life you want, and reducing your pain along the way. The best part is that the more you work your program, the better you'll feel.

The program is structured in three phases:

1. Phase 1: The Humor Festival

2. Phase 2: Bathe in Happy Chemicals

3. Phase 3: Explore Life-Enhancing Activities

Phase 1: The Humor Festival

To start off strong, inject humor into each day. It's as refreshing as a tall glass of lemonade on a hot afternoon. To hold your own humor-based film festival, think back to the films, TV shows, and podcasts that have tickled your funny bone. Many of these shows are available on YouTube or through streaming services. Due to the magic of a smartphone or tablet, you can access humor away from home when you're on the go.

A humor film festival soothes flare-ups and provides an emotional lift. My film festival concept came in handy when I had to taper off the medication Neurontin. I was determined to discontinue the medication because it caused intense itching throughout my body that was driving me crazy.

While I tapered down, I was hit with a severe case of insomnia and couldn't even achieve my usual paltry three hours of sleep. My favorite meditation tapes didn't help me nod off. I was desperately searching for a distraction from the intense itching and lack of sleep when I remembered we had a collection of funny 1990s *Seinfeld* episodes. That helped me to ignore my discomfort and got me to laugh through sleepless nights.

Phase 2: Bathe in Happy Chemicals

Remember the "runner's high" I mentioned that results from sustained exercise? That sense of well-being is the result of activating the neurotransmitter serotonin. This neurotransmitter is only one of the over 100 types of these chemicals in your body.[58] They're major players and help control:

- Heartbeat and blood pressure

- Breathing

- Muscle movements

- Digestion, hunger, and thirst

- Hormone regulation

- Sleeping, healing, and aging

- Stress response

- Thoughts, memory, learning, and feelings

---

58   Dale Purves et al., "Chapter 6: Neurotransmitters," in *Neuroscience*, 2nd ed. (Sunderland, MA: Sinauer Associates, 2001), https://www.ncbi.nlm.nih.gov/books/NBK10795/.

- Responses to senses (what you see, hear, feel, touch and taste)

Each one of these chemicals can be stimulated by performing different types of actions. That's right, you can harness your personal neurotransmitters to help reduce your discomfort. Here's a shortcut for you: scientists have labeled four specific neurotransmitters "happiness chemicals," and the more you stimulate them, the better you feel.

Here are the happy four:

1. Dopamine

2. Oxytocin

3. Serotonin

4. Endorphins

Dopamine is considered the reward chemical. Think about the wonderful buzz you get when you complete a task, cross off something on your to-do list, or eat a favorite meal. That positive feeling is due to the rush of dopamine.

Many people have heard of the love chemical, oxytocin. This chemical is released in the mother's body while giving birth, nursing, and engaging in nurturing their child. It can also occur while playing with a pet, hugging a friend, giving or receiving a compliment, or listening to music that triggers memories of happy times.

Serotonin, the feel-good mood stabilizer chemical, is the one athletes often mention since it elevates their moods. Getting moderate to intense levels of exercise increases serotonin's production. This chemical is important because it reduces anxiety and assists in achieving emotional balance. Research is finding that it aids in wound healing and increases pain tolerance. Walking in nature and meditating also stimulate the release of this chemical.[59]

Endorphins, the last of the mighty four, act as the body's natural painkiller and stress reducer. To stimulate endorphins, all it takes is things like laughter, exercise, the smell of essential oils, indulging in creative pursuits, or getting a taste of dark chocolate.

To remember how to stimulate my happy chemicals, I created a program that I christened my D.O.S.E. Program (the acronym represents the four happy chemicals). This program makes sure that my clients and I receive a healthy dose of each chemical throughout each day to dampen down pain and improve our overall quality of life.

Here's how it works.

We're the director of our own movie. Our cast consists of the four happy chemicals. We get to use the actions we take to decide who gets stage time. Is your pain stealing center stage? Cue the endorphins to enter the scene by watching comedy. Feeling down in the dumps? Summon oxytocin by listening to music. Need motivation? Complete a simple self-care task such as changing out of your PJs or taking a bath. Wanting a "runner's high"? Cast serotonin as your star by employing sustained exercise like a brisk walk.

Here's a cheat sheet for how to get a "D.O.S.E" throughout the day to reduce your discomfort.

Dopamine (Reward)

- Exercise (walk, swim, bike, dance, do yoga).

- Enjoy favorite foods.

---

59   Annamarya Scaccia, "Everything You Need to Know About Serotonin," Healthline, April 17, 2023, https://www.healthline.com/health/mental-health/serotonin.

- Complete a task.

- Perform self-care activities.

- Engage in romantic intimacy or cuddling.

Oxytocin (Love)

- Meditate.

- Play with a pet or entertain a child.

- Hug family and friends.

- Smile and give a compliment.

- Listen to music.

- Relax with a massage.

Serotonin (Feel-Good Mood Stabilizer)

- Exercise (walk, swim, bike, dance, do yoga).

- Eat foods rich in probiotics (miso, kimchi, sourdough, and sauerkraut).

- Meditate.

- Get at least 15 minutes of sunlight.

- Walk in nature.

Endorphin (Painkiller)

- Exercise (walk, swim, bike, dance, do yoga).

- Eat dark chocolate.

- Watch a comedy.

- Smell essential oils or lightly scented candles.

Phase 3: Explore Life-Enhancing Activities

The following strategies are not only accessible, but they can also be budget-friendly. Pick and choose based on personal preference or what brings you joy.

Waves of Wellness: Healing with Aquatic Exercise

Many opening scenes in movies show a swimmer gliding through water. Bubbles float from the swimmer's mouth as the camera follows the person in this magical world. This opening foreshadows the character's upcoming journey and provides a beautiful visual appeal. The imagery not only sets the narrative tone but mirrors the calming benefits of water, such as lowering heart rate and increasing a sense of tranquility.[60]

Exercising in water can be incredibly beneficial, as the buoyancy of the water reduces the force of stress on the joints. This is helpful for people who suffer from arthritis or other painful conditions and those recovering from injuries involving the back, knees, feet, or hips.

Many recreation departments and sports facilities offer aquatic therapy sessions. There's a natural resistance created by moving in water that helps comfortably strengthen muscles in the core, legs, and arms. Water walking is a gentler alternative to water-based aerobics.

Here are disadvantages to water exercises:

- **Sensitivity to chemicals used in the pool** can cause itchy skin and irritate eyes. Some people find showering immediately afterward reduces these problems.

- **Swimmer's ear** is an infection caused by bacteria. The chances of

---

60   Kathleen Holder, "What Are the Health Benefits of Viewing Water?" UC Davis, April 21, 2022, https://www.ucdavis.edu/curiosity/blog/what-are-health-benefits-viewing-water.

getting swimmer's ear increase in high-bacteria areas like public pools. It's caused by excessive moisture trapped in the ear that leads to itching, swelling, drainage, and pain. Drying out your ears as soon as you climb out of the pool or shower is a great preventive measure.

- **Water exercise doesn't burn as many calories or build as much muscle** as land workouts, but if you're not able to exercise on land due to joint pain or injury, water is a good alternative.

Healing Through Pet Companionship

Pictures of pets are always favorite posts on social media. They command more likes and hearts than any other type of post. Why? Animals are adorable, cute, and amazing at making their owners feel loved. Lots of research has found that having a pet enriches your life by reducing stress, anxiety, and depression. Companionship with a pet also releases oxytocin.[61]

You don't have to join the war of whether cats or dogs are better to receive benefits from animal companionship. All sorts of animals can improve your life. Researchers have even found that watching fish in an aquarium has health benefits—it lowers your pulse rate and reduces muscle tension.[62]

Here are situations that may make it hard to own a pet:

- Health challenges can make it too taxing to care for an animal.

- Funds can be limited. Food and vet bills can be costly.

- Pets are prohibited in some living situations.

- Someone in the household is allergic or not pro-animal.

---

61 Lawrence Robinson and Jeanne Segal, "The Health and Mood-Boosting Benefits of Pets," HelpGuide.org, https://www.helpguide.org/articles/mental-health/mood-boosting-power-of-dogs.htm.
62 Robinson and Segal, "Benefits of Pets."

Here are ways to experience the benefits of being with an animal without living with them:

- Volunteer at an animal shelter.

- Visit a local aquarium.

- Watch nature shows.

- Join a bird watchers' group.

- Volunteer to walk your neighborhood dogs or any other pets that need exercise.

- Visit wildlife rehabilitation centers.

Music's Healing Embrace

Studies have shown that music, especially the calm and soothing types, can do wonders to quiet the symptoms of chronic pain.[63] Music also plays a big role in reducing stress and anxiety.

Don't believe me? Stealthily switch the radio station to classical music in a car packed with excitable six-year-olds and see how their behavior changes.

Music also creates bonds between people. Have you ever met a stranger and instantly liked them because they had the same taste in music as you?

When I officiate funerals and memorials, I always ask for a list of favorite songs to play. I know these melodies will comfort the loved ones and friends as much as—or even more than—the words that are spoken.

The great benefit of living today is that smartphones, tablets, and computers make music easily accessible. Listening to music that you enjoy triggers

---

63   Elizabeth Scott, "How Music Can Be Therapeutic," Verywell Mind, updated October 13, 2023, https://www.verywellmind.com/how-and-why-music-therapy-is-effective-3145190.

memories like they happened yesterday. That improves your ability to tolerate discomfort. Music is accessible 24/7, and you have the ability to curate music that lifts your mood. Please don't neglect this potent tool.

Garden Magic: The Healing Wonders of Nature's Touch

One of my favorite novels as a child was *The Secret Garden*. I loved reading about the two young children finding the magic and lure of a hidden garden that no one knew about. I can't have been the only one enchanted by the tale because the novel has been made into a major movie at least three times, as long ago as 1919.

People around the world relate to the miracle of nature and its beauty. An overwhelming feeling of awe comes from witnessing the cycle of nature. This can be calming, therapeutic, and fulfilling.

Studies have proven that fresh air and gardening activities such as planting, weeding, watering, and pruning promote relaxation, reduce anxiety, and provide a sense of tranquility. Not only that, but they also tap into a person's creativity and personal style and can be one of the best antidepressants out there. Not to mention that growing vegetables and fruits will improve your diet while reducing food costs![64]

Many cities around the world have established community gardens for their residents. These public plots provide a portion of land for apartment dwellers and others who don't have access to land where they can plant their vegetables, fruits, and flowers.

If gardening's too taxing for you, consider adding house plants to your home environment. House plants can brighten your home and lift your spirits.

---

64   Rebecca Joy Stanborough, "Seed, Soil, and Sun: Discovering the Many Helpful Benefits of Gardening," Healthline, June 17, 2020, https://www.healthline.com/health/healthful-benefits-of-gardening.

They also clear the air of pollutants, so you can consider them as your natural air filters. An inexpensive way to incorporate the gardening experience into your life is to grow herbs and sprout seeds in your kitchen. Another way to enjoy plants is to walk in a forest. Nature's dense collection of plants and trees provides the same benefits as spending time in human-cultivated gardens.

Unleashing Healing Through Expressive Arts

The first time I heard the phrase "expressive arts" in class, I pictured a painter in a smock covered with paint, brush in hand, under a creative frenzy. Given that my stick figures are wiggle lines and my sunsets look more like blobs of orange-and-yellow paint, I figured that this healing modality wasn't for me. When I dug a little deeper out of curiosity, I found out that I was wrong. It could be for me too.

Expressive arts are where you express your emotions and intuition through various mediums. This includes writing and storytelling, films, music, plays, sewing, photography, dance, stringing beads, weaving, and even street art.

Once I understood that my drawing ability didn't matter, it gave me freedom to express myself. I discovered that not only do people find my whimsical gardens unique, but they're also enamored by the handcrafted jewelry I designed in my quest to recover the use of my damaged dominant hand. I first practiced stringing large wooden beads to improve coordination and flexibility. Over time, I graduated to smaller plastic beads and then, finally, to stringing gemstones. My jewelry has a unique look because my design decisions are a result of what my fingers are willing to do at the time I'm creating each piece.

Once, when I was on a chaplaincy visit with a woman receiving her chemo infusion, she noticed the handcrafted bracelet I was wearing. She loved the jewelry and asked if I had another she could buy from me. I removed the bracelet and gave it to her, telling her to consider it a healing gift. Her smile and the rush of oxytocin I experienced launched my practice of sending surprise necklaces, bracelets, and earrings to women facing life-threatening illnesses or difficult family life situations. These women wouldn't have experienced the warmth that comes with knowing someone cares if I'd let my insecurity about being an artist stand in my way.

Another form of expressive arts that targets the neurotransmitters is storytelling. Listening to or even reading a story mentally transports us to another time and place. Our brains are hardwired to synchronize in the moment with those of the storyteller, and our pain has been found to recede when we are listening to or reading stories.

For 14 months during the pandemic, I used storytelling to lift my spirits and those of my Instagram and Facebook followers. Authoring stories about courage stimulated my dopamine, and then responding to the comments left stimulated my oxytocin. Later in the book, you'll read about how this storytelling experience helped me build a social network.

What form of expressive art or favorite hobby speaks to you? Do you enjoy journaling or doodling as you sit through meetings? Perhaps you create amazing entrées or desserts and present them in an eye-catching manner. Or maybe you collect trains, play video games, or enjoy playing bridge. All these activities will improve your quality of life.

Case Study: Sjögren's Syndrome

Last year I was surprised to receive a Zoom invite from my old college friend Jenny. We usually text every couple of months and then hold a marathon phone call every New Year's Day to start the year off right. This Zoom invite was to discuss Jenny's recent diagnosis of Sjögren's syndrome.

Sjögren's Syndrome

Sjögren's syndrome (SS) is another one of those masked mugger autoimmune diseases that lurks in the shadows, then pounces hard, stealing away health. The first time you may realize the impact of the mugging is when one part of your body (like your eyes) and then another part (like your skin) becomes uncomfortably dry. SS first attacks your body's moisture-producing glands. The disease also leads to fatigue. Both muscle and joint pain are common side effects, along with chronic cough, vaginal dryness, and thyroid issues.

SS is difficult to diagnose because its symptoms mimic those of other medical conditions. Since 95% of its victims are women, the symptoms it presents are often attributed to menopause. Younger women afflicted with SS often first attribute the symptoms to medication side effects.

Common complications of SS include dental cavities due to mouth dryness, thrush (a yeast infection in the mouth), and vision problems due to light sensitivity, blurred vision, and corneal damage. SS can also lead to lung disease, kidney problems, digestive issues, and liver dysfunction.

Symptoms

- Dry eyes

- Dry mouth

- Less commonly, joint pain, swollen glands, rashes or dry skin, vaginal dryness, dry cough, and fatigue.

Risk Factors

- Genetics
- Immune dysfunction

- Hormones
- Viral infections

Diagnosis

- Blood tests
- Eye tests
- Imaging
- Biopsy

Treatments

- NSAIDs

- Corticosteroids

- Disease-modifying antirheumatic drugs (DMARDs)

- Biologics

- Prescriptions to treat dry mouth and eyes

- Mindfulness and cognitive behavioral therapy[65]

Jenny—a tall, slender blond—and I first met in a health social issues college class in the 1970s. We immediately became friends over the fact that we were not in pursuit of our MRS degrees. At that time, a woman's choice of career included being a teacher, librarian, social worker, nurse, or flight attendant. Jenny chose to major in nursing. I'd always been interested in medicine, but I was squeamish about death, so I chose to major in health education and social work. That 18-year-old me would've been amazed to hear that, 29 years later, I became a chaplain who regularly visits hospice patients and officiates at funerals and memorials.

Our friendship continued over the years. I've always appreciated Jenny's dry sense of humor and the fact we've offered one another a safe harbor. When I was diagnosed with CRPS, she taught me the inexpensive trick of coating my skin with Maalox to prevent skin rashes from the TENS unit's electrodes. And when she was diagnosed with breast cancer, she shared her fears with me

---

65   "Sjogren's Syndrome," Mayo Clinic, August 2, 2022, https://www.mayoclinic.org/diseases-conditions/sjogrens-syndrome/diagnosis-treatment/drc-20353221.

to empower her to keep a brave front for her family and coworkers.

I was now looking into the face of a 70-year-old friend whose wrinkles and gray hair melted away as soon as she smiled. She had called herself a bean-stalk in college since her 5'9" height put her head and shoulders above other women. Back in the day, I had envied her long, straight, blond hair that hung halfway down her back. During college, I'd carefully blow-dry my long, thick, black hair to remove my curls. Much to my dismay, my curls always returned whenever San Francisco's fog rolled in. Now that we're in our seventh decade, we both have short hairstyles.

We had a brief catch-up about family and friends, and then I asked her how retirement was going.

"During the pandemic, I answered the call-out for retired nurses and realized I missed nursing. Last year I joined a group of other semi-retired nurses to provide services to families in our local shelter.

"Our community converted an old motel to house the homeless near the rail line. This allows the residents to get to their jobs and medical appointments. Each family has their own unit instead of being housed dormitory style."

"Wow, that sounds wonderful."

She nodded, unable to hold back her smile. "I love making a real difference."

"Are you providing basic nursing care?"

She looked at me for a moment before saying, "Many of our residents need help with their mental health issues and substance use disorders." Her voice had grown sad as she talked about the challenges. "I spend much of my time assessing their needs and referring them to support agencies." She added with a smile, "The best part is working with the children. We see that they have breakfast and lunch boxes filled with nutritious food before they go to school."

It was sad to envision young kids spending time in a homeless shelter.

"I'm sure the shelter appreciates your involvement."

She let out a disappointed sigh. "I love it, but I've had to step back because of my SS diagnosis."

I gasped. "When were you diagnosed with it?"

"I went for an eye exam, and my optometrist noted my eyes were extremely dry and said I should use eye drops four times a day." She tipped her chin up with amusement. "You know me, so you won't be surprised that I quipped that I was already using lozenges for my dry mouth and shoving lubricating suppositories up my private parts. I thought the doc's look came from him being a prude, but instead he said that if I'm also dry and irritated in those areas, I needed to have my internist run tests."

Optometrists are often at the forefront for detecting a host of medical conditions, including heart disease, high blood pressure, high cholesterol, lupus, multiple sclerosis, and rheumatoid arthritis, as well as spotting possible threats for stroke and Graves' disease. The reason for this is that all these health conditions cause observable changes in the eye.

"That's not something you want to hear during an eye exam," I told my good friend. I shifted in my chair to appear calm as I digested her troubling news.

"Oh, Bonnie, they put me through so much testing, and then I heard I had SS." She shook her head as though wanting to shake the news away. "It's so overwhelming to think I have another fight ahead of me. I thought I was free of this stuff when my cancer went into remission."

"I'm so sorry."

She closed her eyes, taking a deep breath, still upset.

"How're you doing now that you've been diagnosed?"

She shrugged. "The meds calm my symptoms, but they're making me put on weight. My vision is still bad. My eye doc thinks the eye drops will help. I hope they work so I can keep driving."

I leaned forward with my chin resting on my hand. "Remember when I wanted to teach a stress management class to inner-city second graders and thought that my CRPS was robbing me of my ability to help them?"

She used a tissue to wipe the corner of her eyes.

"You said," I continued, "that if I showed up at their class every Friday afternoon, it would be a highlight of their day even if I wasn't 100%."

Jenny gave a slow smile. "You're right. No, I mean, I was right. I should listen to myself."

Part of her listening to herself was her getting back on a schedule of volunteering at the shelter and adding humor and play into her day. For her, that meant using puppets when she interacted with the shelter's children.

At our next meeting, the screen opened up with Jenny laughing as she wiggled her fingers at me. She had a farm animal on each finger—a pig, chicken, cow, donkey, horse, duck, lamb, goose, turkey, and goat. She shared tales about what a success these finger puppets were at lifting her spirits and everyone else's at the shelter.

My old wisecracking friend was on the mend and ready to add more happy chemicals into her life by using the D.O.S.E. method. In our later meetings, we explored her possibilities for using expressive arts, gardening, and music. She chose to plant a garden at the shelter and took it to a new level when she convinced local nurseries to donate planters and plants.

Kids and their parents attended a class put on by the nursery's head gardener where they learned how to amend the soil and break up the root ball of each plant before planting. Everyone was encouraged to work in the vegetable garden and took turns selecting their favorite music to play as they watered and weeded.

For an art project, Jenny encouraged staff and residents to collect stones the kids could paint. This became a great public relations activity. Businesses on the street suddenly found inspirational hand-painted rocks in their landscape instead of litter.

The local newspaper caught wind of the changes at the shelter and ran a story about the mayor and business owners supporting the facility that helped people get back on their feet. The article was accompanied by photos showing the thriving garden beds decorated with the painted rocks.

Jenny's involvement with the shelter gave her the opportunity to see how simple strategies could not only assist her in dealing with the emotional impact of SS but could also improve the lives of families coping with the stress of homelessness.

If you have any doubt that you will be able to improve your health by adopting self-care strategies in your home environment, please give yourself the gift of consistently practicing a few of the activities described in this chapter. I guarantee that by combining these activities with your current treatment program, you'll improve your life. It won't make your pain vanish, but you'll have effective coping tools.

In the next chapter, you'll learn how lifestyle medicine can improve your current health and prevent or reverse type 2 diabetes, hypertension, arthritis, and other lifestyle illnesses.

REMEMBER:

- There are many affordable and accessible self-care strategies that can improve your quality of life.

- Self-care strategies create positive changes in your neural pathways that can lead to healing opportunities.

- Exploring self-care strategies can help you find new areas of interest and undiscovered talents in your life.

- Humor, music, and remembering to utilize D.O.S.E. can minimize a flare-up and help you cope with chronic issues.

CHAPTER 9

Essential Nourishment for Healing

♥

"Let thy food be thy medicine"

—ATTRIBUTED TO HIPPOCRATES, PHYSICIAN AND TEACHER

P ain is a silent thief zapping away our joy, our energy, our mobility, our productivity, and our relationships and sometimes affecting our ability to think. It can chisel away our sense of competence.

My self-image certainly took a hit as I dealt with my pain. It ate at me that I didn't put a smile on my husband's face very often. I lacked the ability to be the energetic mom I longed to be for my son. I also hated that I had put time and money into pursuing an advanced degree, but my health only allowed me to volunteer for a few hours a week at my son's school.

My days were spent not measuring up when one day, as I was lying on my couch resting, a documentary on the ancient practice of kintsugi, the art of being broken, popped up. In this practice, which dates back to the 15th century, an artisan mends broken pottery with gold or other precious metals to transform the broken pottery into something stronger than it was before. In the tradition of this art, the artisan doesn't disguise or hide the broken pieces. They celebrate the beauty of damage that comes with life. The scars are transformed to symbolize resilience, healing, and the beauty of imperfection.

As I watched the show, I saw the parallels between kintsugi and my strategies that strove to put me back together. Like the golden seams that mended broken pottery, my own healing strategies honored the damage that I had and continued to strengthen me and put me back together stronger.

My strategies forced me to acknowledge the very depth of my brokenness, the pain and impact it had on my form, and then to lovingly see the beauty and art it had to offer. After seeing the miracle of the broken, I zealously used my strategies, determination, and self-love to mend using research material, my schooling, and intuition. Or, in other words, my knowledge was what I used to create the gold, the bonding agent, that I was using to rebuild my body, mind, and soul into a stronger, more resilient version of myself.

Each scar, each challenge, each betrayal, and each sorrow became a symbol of my journey that I'd survived. Thinking about this, I now saw magnificent beauty in my personal journey. We each have the ability to grasp our past and present pain and then shift into celebrating the profound richness life has to offer us. Our wounds, our scars, and our pains are our art that can become our personal masterpiece.

To craft our individual masterpiece of our body, it's important to give the body the best material to build and construct with. Part of our gold, if we continue with the kintsugi art metaphor, is the nutrition we pour into our bodies.

When we talk about nutrition, the conversation often leads to weight. Before you groan, I know it's rare for people to be satisfied with their weight. The topic is a minefield for people living with chronic pain. The medications we take, supposedly to give us hope, barely touch our agony, and too many times add pounds while causing incredibly uncomfortable side effects.

Added to this, many patients don't move or exercise because it hurts even to breathe. The combination of added pounds and the inability to keep our bodies toned can result in our clothes becoming snug. It's hard to look in the mirror at our pain, weight, and the ravages our conditions take.

A downward spiral can easily happen when the doctor who prescribed our medications tells us to diet or accept the weight gain as part of the condition. At this point, many patients report that going to their doctor's visits becomes a painful guilt and shamefest.

Uncomfortable Truth About Our Health

When we're being flooded with pain, it's hard to think about anything but getting out of it. It's especially hard to want to tackle the mountain called "diet." After all, the word "diet" has the word "die" in it for a reason! But thinking about it, if it's possible to relieve the pain in our backs, hips, knees, and other joints by switching our food choices, wouldn't it be worth it?

Not convinced yet? I wasn't. When the surgeon who promised to end my suffering through surgery saw me for a postoperative appointment, he wasn't happy about the intensified burning sensations and spasms throughout my body. Plus, I'd developed TMJ from clenching my jaw due to my growing agony.

I stood in the exam room, unable to sit anymore. It had taken over an hour to reach the surgeon's office. While I gave him an update about my symptoms, I leaned against the exam table, shifting my weight.

He reached for my flaccid dominant left hand and frowned to find it swollen and red. He continued to scowl as he wrote on a prescription pad. The prescription was for off-label use of Prozac, a new selective serotonin reuptake inhibitor that had been introduced the year before.

"Maybe this will help with the burning," he muttered.

I took the piece of paper from his pudgy fingers.

"Perhaps if you lost five or ten pounds you'd feel better," he added, giving me a disapproving frown.

I stared at him, stopping myself from telling him he'd feel better if he stopped smoking and lying to his patients. Despite myself, shame washed over me. I'm short with a curvy figure, and even in my competitive swimming days, my muscular build never reflected the slender body of a fashion model.

I shouldn't be made to feel bad for my body shape—ever, and especially not after he had ruined my body to the level he had. Clearly, I was a diagnostic code to him, and he had no understanding of what he had done to me, nor did he care.

"You may be a candidate for a spinal cord stimulator, or SCS, that acts like an internal TENS unit." He moved toward the door.

I was never going to undergo any further invasive medical interventions. None. Wouldn't be happening. My days of being an experiment were over. Nor was I going to take advice from someone who had no idea what it was like to live in pain. Instead, I was going to stick to what was working—focusing on the pillars of health. That meant focusing on nutrition, not weight. Frankly, at that time, I was so miserable that I couldn't care less about how I looked; all I wanted was to stop hurting.

At first, my anger kept me going. I wanted to show that doctor that healthy lifestyle behaviors were more powerful than his knife. I switched the fats in my diet to plant-based omega-3s. That change reduced the inflammation in my body. I increased the quantity of grains and vegetables I ate, which trimmed off the 10 pounds suggested by the surgeon and improved my blood pressure. Despite all that, the CRPS symptoms remained a constant. I vowed to never see a quality-of-life-destroying doctor again.

In 2000 I experienced a horrible flare-up after enjoying a prime rib dinner. My hands swelled, and I experienced stiffness in my joints and increased spasms throughout my body. That was a flashing red light telling me to stop eating all meat.

Avoiding all types of meat improved my digestion. I never experienced that type of flare-up again. This was the first time I saw that not only could food impact weight and heart health and cause type 2 diabetes, but it could also increase or decrease aches.

I was on an intense crusade to improve my overall health and didn't stop by just cutting out meat. At this point in my healing journey, my CRPS wasn't only causing me pain, but it affected the circulation in my left arm and hand. This made that area feel icy cold and made my fingers swell.

When I read that consuming oil can temporarily compromise the function of the endothelial cells that form the interior surface of our blood vessels and can affect inflammation, I said goodbye to all types of oil. That's right, no oil for me, not even olive oil. The outcome? I experienced less swelling in my hand.[66]

I don't miss oil at all, especially since I learned that I can easily sauté my

---

66   Caldwell Esselstyn, *Prevent and Reverse Heart Disease: The Revolutionary, Scientifically Proven, Nutrition-Based Cure* (New York: Penguin Group, 2008).

food in water or broth. My salads are always dressed with flavored balsamic vinegar or oil-free hummus. When I make baked goods, I substitute sugar-free applesauce for oil.

A few months later, after I made these changes to my diet, I had lunch with a friend.

When I placed my order, he looked at me with a frown. "So you've become a vegan?"

I had ordered a salad without chicken or shredded cheese dressed with flavored balsamic vinegar and sunflower seeds. When I thought about what I'd been eating for the past few days and weeks, it was obvious that my choices could be labeled "vegan."

That night, I dove into researching the vegan diet. My friend's guess had been right. I had strayed into a vegan diet. No pork or shellfish (easy, since I'm Jewish). I had stopped eating fish years before because of an allergy. I'd already given up eating chicken, turkey, and eggs after I began rescuing parrots in the 1990s. Dairy was out too due to my lactose intolerance, and I never used honey because I found it too sweet.

Going vegan is a popular choice among those suffering health issues, and some do it to prevent animal suffering. Others join in to slow down global warming.[67] This approach isn't for everyone, but it worked for me, so I stayed with it.

Upon further research, I learned that I'd gone beyond becoming vegan. Since I don't use oil, my food style is referred to as "whole-food plant-based no oil," or WFPBNO. Within six months of eating this way, my blood pressure

---

67   Ker Than, "Could Going Vegan Help Reduce Greenhouse Gas Emissions?" *Stanford Earth Matters Magazine*, February 2, 2022, https://sustainability.stanford.edu/news/could-going-vegan-help-reduce-greenhouse-gas-emissions.

returned to normal. I was able to get off my hypertension medication. My tight clothes felt comfortable, and I ate an unlimited quantity of vegetables, grains, fruits, potatoes, and legumes rather than being on a portion-controlled diet.

The foods I was eating had less calorie density (they were lower in calories per gram) than animal protein. Also, making sure not to consume anything with added refined sugar ensured I could eat until I felt full, knowing I could easily maintain my weight loss. My delicious entrées included plant-based lasagna, enchilada casserole, chili, and curries. My desserts included sweet baked goods created without sugar or oil.

This works well at home, but out in the community, I'm careful to be on the lookout to avoid frozen vegan entrées stocked in grocery stores that include preservatives, fats, and sugars. This goes for restaurants too. Sometimes the touted vegan meal listed on a menu relies on added fats and salt to make it more enjoyable. Some plant-based people enjoy this type of meal every now and then, but with my condition, I'm vigilant to protect my circulatory system. I usually order a huge salad and a plain baked potato that I douse with salsa or the smoked hickory balsamic vinegar that I carry when I'm dining out.

By eating this way, I'm receiving all the protein and nutrients my body needs. This curbs my appetite and leaves me full. The only added supplement needed on a plant-predominant diet (meaning a diet focusing on plants) is vitamin B12.

Although this way of eating has given me my health back, sometimes when I dine with groups of people and order a plant and grain entrée without cheese, I'll hear someone say, "Why don't you live a little and enjoy yourself?"

I always share that the way I eat helps control my neurological condition so that I don't have to depend on opioids. This stirs people's curiosity, and I'm often contacted later for more information about the possible link between food and their health issues. I explain that fried foods and foods high in added sugar, refined carbohydrates, alcohol, and meat cause inflammation in the body.

Growing restless during the pandemic, I hunted YouTube for plant-based cooking shows to jazz up my meal options. As I conducted this search, not only did I stumble onto yummy healthy recipes, but YouTube's algorithm kicked in. It started suggesting "lifestyle medicine" podcasts that explored how our daily life choices affect our health.

These podcasts were packed with great information and fascinated me. While listening to them, I discovered that lifestyle medicine had received a make-over by scientists. The traditional four pillars of health I had learned about in the 1970s had been modernized to include six pillars. The current pillars:

1. Nutrition

2. Movement

3. Avoiding damaging substances

4. Managing stress

5. Improving sleep

6. Maintaining positive social connections

Digging deeper into the world of lifestyle medicine, I discovered that in 2004, the American College of Lifestyle Medicine (ACLM) was established to advocate for how lifestyle choices can influence disease prevention and help manage chronic health issues.

After working for over four decades to encourage healthier lifestyles, I was deeply moved that I wasn't on a mission alone. With a membership including physicians, dieticians, nurses, health educators, pain coaches like me, and students, ACLM represents an entire community dedicated to this growing movement.

In the blink of an eye, I joined up to learn the most current health information braniac scientists had discovered. All of us health professionals meet a few times a month to review the latest findings and to discuss how we can influence people to adopt healthy behaviors. This professional connection continues to provide me with valuable information for my health webinars and in-person workshops.

I was excited during an ACLM meeting to learn about an opportunity to update my credentials. I jumped on it and enrolled in Cornell University's T. Colin Campbell Center for Nutrition Studies, where I earned a plant-based nutrition certificate.

In the earlier chapters, I shared personalized strategies I used to achieve the pain-free existence I enjoy today. In this chapter and the next five, we'll explore other ways to feel better by using the principles from the modernized lifestyle medicine pillars. Today, at 72, I continue to flourish by using these healthy behaviors as my North Star to support my health.

One of the healthy behaviors you can consider using as part of your kintsugi gold to help you mend your body is focusing on a plant-predominant diet.

Many clients I work with are only concerned at first with feeling better. I tell them they will if they avoid ultra-processed foods and increase their fruits, vegetables, and grains in their food program. I always caution patients with celiac disease and Hashimoto's thyroid disease to avoid gluten.[68]

Remember, it's about improving your health and should be considered a food plan and not a restricted diet. Each person can explore which tweaks in their diet will help them. Diet is a crucial factor in neuroplasticity. Healthy foods improve cognitive function and prevent age-related brain diseases that result in cognitive decline. Nutrition also helps the brain to change and adapt.

A good way to design your food plan is to figure out if your food choices are health-enhancing or health-detracting.[69]

Health-Enhancing Foods

- Vegetables

- Fruits (Avoid if you're fructose intolerant or have other conditions that react badly to natural sugar.)

- Legumes (Unless you have stomach issues with them. Sometimes it takes the body time to adjust to digesting legumes.)

- Grains (If you have celiac disease or are allergic to gluten, avoid grains that have gluten.)

- Nuts and seeds (If you have a lot of allergies, get evaluated to establish which ones are safe for you.)

- If you choose to include meat in your diet, it should be less than 7% fat.

Health-Detracting Foods

68 "Hashimoto's Thyroiditis Diet: Best & Worst Food List," Baptist Health, February 28, 2021, https://www.baptisthealth.com/blog/family-health/hashimoto-s-thyroiditis-diet-best-worst-food-list.

69 "Heart-Healthy Diet: 8 Steps to Prevent Heart Disease," Mayo Clinic, April 28, 2022, https://www.mayoclinic.org/diseases-conditions/heart-disease/in-depth/heart-healthy-diet/art-20047702.

- Saturated fats

- Processed meats

- Salty foods (Always follow your doctor's orders if your health condition requires more salt.)

- High-fat dairy

- Added sugar

Simple Steps to Improve Your Nutrition

1. Eat more low-calorie, nutrient-rich foods like vegetables and fruits.

2. Eat smaller portions of high-calorie foods.

3. Cut high-calorie, high-sodium foods.

4. Select whole grains unless you're allergic or have celiac or Hashimoto's thyroid disease.

5. Limit unhealthy fats.

6. Choose low-fat protein sources like legumes, tofu, sprouted grains, quinoa, nuts, and seeds.

7. Substitute dairy milk with plant-based milk.

8. Limit or reduce salt by using herbs and spices.

9. Start your day with whole-grain cereal, plant milk, and fresh fruit.

10. Schedule at least one fully plant-based dinner every week.

11. Steam, roast, or bake rather than fry food.

12. Watch cooking shows to learn how to make nutrient-rich and heart-healthy treats.

Out of the list I just mentioned above, I have clients start with reducing their intake of sugar and unhealthy fats. Scientists have found a strong connection between consuming sugar and unhealthy fats and a reduction in the brain's ability to adapt to change. Incorporating healthy fats and antioxidants in one's diet has been shown to bolster neuroplasticity and cognitive health.[70]

As you add more fruits, vegetables, and grains into your diet, it's important to go slow and listen to your body to discover if a specific food aggravates your condition or causes other problems like gastrointestinal issues, skin eruptions, or swelling. The way to know which food is causing the issue is by adding only one new food in at a time.

No one diet is perfect for all bodies. I transitioned to my way of eating because I listened to what my body told me. There are many vegetables that don't agree with me. I avoid them and concentrate on getting my fiber and micronutrients from the vegetables and fruits I can easily digest.

The other challenge of changing what we eat is eating with other people. Food plays a huge role in holiday celebrations, weddings, and childhood-to-adulthood rites of passage. Our ties to our heritage are represented by our food choices. Unfortunately, food today has been processed using sugar, fat, and sodium to a level that is injurious to our health. Being aware of these changes can help you better balance the consumption of celebratory food with your healing food choices.

---

70   "Diet and Neuroplasticity: How What You Eat Affects Your Brain," NeuroLaunch, July 13, 2022, archived November 26, 2022, at the Wayback Machine, https://web.archive.org/web/20221126080806/https://neurolaunch.com/diet-and-neuroplasticity-how-what-you-eat-affects-your-brain/.

Case Study: Osteoarthritis

♥

"The shoemaker's children have no shoes."

—PROVERB

It wasn't until the pandemic that my then-78-year-old husband reached out to me for help with a flare-up of osteoarthritis in his back and hands. Osteoarthritis (OA) is the most common type of arthritis and affects over 32.5 million U.S. adults.[71] If you ask a room full of people if they know anyone with osteoarthritis, almost everyone's hand will shoot up. If they don't have an achy knee, shoulder, hands, or neck, then one of their parents or grandparents is living with the aches and pain of OA.

Osteoarthritis

Another label for OA is degenerative joint disease. This refers to the wearing down of the protective cartilage that cushions the ends of the bones. This degeneration usually develops slowly and becomes worse over time. It can cause pain, stiffness, and swelling. Some people experience reduced function and disability and are no longer able to carry out daily living tasks.[72]

OA can damage all joints, but it most often affects the joints in the hands, knees, and hips.

Symptoms

- Pain

---

71   "Osteoarthritis," Centers for Disease Control and Prevention, last updated June 12, 2023, https://www.cdc.gov/arthritis/basics/osteoarthritis.htm.

72   "Osteoarthritis," Centers for Disease Control and Prevention.

- Stiffness

- Decreased range of motion (flexibility)

- Swelling[73]

Risk Factors

- Joint injury or overuse (such as sports injuries or repetitive knee bending or hand and wrist movements on the job)

- Age: Risk increases with age

- Obesity: Causes stress on the weight-bearing joints like the knees and hips

- Genetics: More prevalent in families with a history of OA. People with hand OA are more prone to develop knee OA.[74]

- Certain metabolic diseases: Diabetes and hemochromatosis (too much iron in the body)

- Bone deformities: Birth defects involving malformed joints or defective cartilage

- Hypermobility[75]

Diagnosis

- Review of symptoms

- Physical exam

- X-rays

- Lab tests[76]

73   "Osteoarthritis," Centers for Disease Control and Prevention.
74   "Osteoarthritis," Centers for Disease Control and Prevention.
75   Chenhui Cai et al. "Interplay Between Iron Overload and Osteoarthritis: Clinical Significance and Cellular Mechanisms." *Frontiers in Cell and Developmental Biology* 9 (January 14, 2022): 817104. doi:10.3389/fcell.2021.817104
76   "Osteoarthritis," Centers for Disease Control and Prevention.

Treatments

- Increased physical activity

- Physical therapy with muscle-strengthening exercises

- Weight loss

- Medications, including over-the-counter pain relievers and prescription drugs

- Supportive devices such as canes or crutches and mouth guards

- Surgery if other options haven't been effective[77]

- Moving to a warmer climate

- Mindfulness and CBT to manage depression and sleep disturbances that can result from the pain and disability of OA

My "never going to retire" husband Len was offered a wonderful deal—an early retirement option given to long-time employees due to a company reorganization. He had been programming for 56 years and loved his work. The idea of not working was daunting.

The offer meant he'd stop working in six months but would continue receiving a full salary for another year. If he took it, his early retirement checks would stop right before his 80th birthday. Knowing that this was an amazing deal, he accepted the offer and wrote "137 days" on his office whiteboard.

As the numbers dwindled, his behavior shifted. The changes were subtle—things like his usual stash of Oreos, which had usually lasted a month, suddenly needing to be replenished every few days. For the first time ever, he thumped up and down the hallways at two in the morning, unable to sleep. The most concerning change happened when he announced, "I can't seem to

---

77 "Osteoarthritis," Centers for Disease Control and Prevention.

concentrate on programming."

We discussed that for a while, then he asked me if I'd sit in his office with him as he talked through each programming step. I couldn't think of anything more boring, but he almost never asked for help. Sitting beside him, I noticed that, between tapping the keys, he massaged his fingers, rubbed his back and neck, and squirmed in his chair.

When he paused from work, I asked, "Something wrong with your fingers?"

"They're stiff."

A telltale sign that his stress was playing havoc with his OA.

After he finished his project, I asked him if he was open to some suggestions.

He leaned back in his chair and crossed his arms. "Like what?"

"Your OA symptoms are worsening."

"How can you tell?" he grumbled.

I went over his symptoms.

He frowned.

"There're things you can do to lessen them."

His brow knitted. "I'm not a client."

"Want out of pain?" I shot back.

"Fine, tell me what you're busting at the seams to say."

"Well," I dove in, "there're little things you can do to feel more comfortable. First off, you can elevate your desk to a standing position a couple of times a day. That'd relieve the stress on your back."

"Fine," he said.

"You can set your phone alarm to remind you to use heat and massage to calm down your swollen joints."

"Okay."

I placed a bottle of over-the-counter anti-inflammatories next to his computer.

He scowled. "I'm not taking pills."

"These pills will combat the enemy that's causing the inflammation in your angry joints."

He stood and left the room, only to return a few minutes later with a glass of water that he set down next to the pills.

Game on.

The next morning, after feeding him his special breakfast treat of French toast and chicken apple sausages, I tackled the villain that I suspected was giving him stress: anxiety. This can be a tough topic with men who believe anxiety is for wimps.

"You know, your difficulty in concentrating may be a sign that you're anxious about your upcoming retirement," I said tentatively.

He plunked down his fork on his empty plate. "How can I be anxious? You don't see me breaking out in a cold sweat, do you?"

He had a career of playing Mr. Cool-and-Collected, a reputation that he earned from his calm guidance during middle-of-the-night calls when a critical system was crashing. I found his steadiness impressive.

"Let me review the symptoms of anxiety, and you tell me if any of them fit."

He crossed his arms over his chest but nodded for me to go on.

"Change in sleep pattern."

"Check."

"Easily distracted."

"Check."

"Change in appetite."

"Check, again."

And so it went as he heard familiar symptoms he was experiencing. Knowing he's a consummate tech guy, I suggested an app (unwindinganxiety.com) that could teach him how to deal with stress and conquer his anxiety. He added it to his arsenal of arthritis-fighting weapons, which also included heating and massaging his fingers.

A few months after he made these behavior changes, we left our town for the first time since the pandemic hit. The destination was Yosemite National Park, our state's treasure. It's in central California, three hours from our Dublin home.

I'd promised a dying high school classmate that I'd officiate her memorial in the park, but to this point, fulfilling that promise had been derailed by the pandemic. The weather was a comfortable 68 degrees with a clear blue sky.

The traffic was light as we passed through the quiet small towns.

As I drove, I stole a covert glance to admire my tall, silver-haired husband's newly shorn locks. I had spiffed him up with a pandemic haircut the day before for the day's event. I had used YouTube to guide me through an Ivy League cut, which is a longer version of the crew cut.

"Not bad, but don't give up your day job," I thought to myself.

He was oblivious to my attention, listening to his Unwinding Anxiety app with earbuds.

As we drove up to Yosemite's main entrance gate, I mused to myself about how amazing it is that portable high-tech apps can offer emotional support on the go. I also took in the protected majestic views that haven't changed since President Theodore Roosevelt and the naturalist John Muir visited the park way back in 1903. The earthy smells of the forest filled the air as we made our way to gather at the trailhead for the memorial. Standing among the pine cones and curious squirrels and deer, I recited my classmate's favorite poem, "Remember Me," fulfilling her final wish.

She was on my mind as we drove home that evening. We'd been good friends in high school, but we had lost touch over the years. We had reconnected in 2017 when I had showed up at a barbeque hosted by an old high school classmate. While we caught up on what had happened over the past years, she had me rolling on the floor laughing as she told stories about owning a trucking company and dealing with all sorts of characters.

She had a big and bold personality, and even though all her neighbors viewed her as having a huge and caring heart, she could successfully deal with the rough-and-tumble of bidding for highway contracts with the state. If I had to choose one word to describe her, it would be "courageous."

As I thought about her, Len had grown quiet. I could tell by the way he shifted in his seat that his OA was bothering him a lot. That night, I tossed and turned, thinking about his health. By the time morning arrived, I had a plan.

His pandemic weight gain played havoc with his osteoarthritis. That meant I had to enter a land where no one likes to venture—challenging a man who grew up with meat and mashed potatoes and gravy, vegetables just a garnish on his plate. Desserts were rich puddings, Oreos, or his all-time favorite, pie à la mode.

He'd never been interested in eating plant-based meals, so I always prepared two different meals for us. Secretly, I took to reducing the salt and fat in his favorite entrées. Probably out of guilt, he reduced his own consumption of rich desserts, choosing instead to keep a stash of his cookies in his office.

But now he was hurting, and I knew his joints would be happier if he transitioned to an anti-inflammatory whole-food plant-based no oil diet. Since I consider myself the pain police, always on the prowl to arrest it, I acted.

That morning, instead of preparing Len's usual cold cereal with milk and banana, I prepared a hearty bowl of oatmeal and fruit and set up my iPad in the breakfast nook so he could view the documentary *The Game Changers*. It's my go-to documentary when I discuss a plant-focused diet with men. It features elite athletes who transition to a plant-based diet and highlights scientific studies extolling the benefits of switching out animal protein, including dairy, from your diet.

Len watched the video, saying nothing, but after eating the oatmeal, he put his dirty bowl in the sink and said, "I'll try it for a week."

"Mean it?"

"Sure."

"Then go grab your coat."

"Why?"

"We have a month's worth of your frozen 'healthy' meat entrées to give to our divorced and widowed neighbors."

He shook his head. "I have some programming to do. Have fun."

He hated the idea of being stuck in small talk conversations with the neighbors, which was absolutely fine. It gave me more time to chat, not worrying about him feeling trapped and wanting to get home.

Surprising us both, his transition to a WFPBNO vegan lifestyle was no problem. All he had to do was show up at the table three times a day. Oh, yeah, and give up his cookies.

For me, the challenge was to cook tantalizing recipes so he wouldn't miss his old food. Within a day of eating this way, he noticed a spike in his energy. By day two, he had stopped his afternoon snacking, claiming he was too full. And, miracle of miracles, after three days, he no longer thought about his hamburgers, french fries, and Cokes. By day five, his lifelong stuffy nose finally cleared up.

Day six, he wanted to learn more of the science behind this new way of eating. He signed up for NutritionFacts.org, a science-based organization's website featuring videos. Each morning, he got up and listened to the latest nutrition study and enthusiastically shared the findings.

On day seven, he said his taste buds were more alive than ever and his belt was looser.

In August, only four months after he had transitioned to his new way of eating, his company held a videoconference-based retirement party for him.

At the last minute, the video went down, and nobody saw that Len had lost 30 pounds. He laughed when somebody said they hoped he didn't turn into a couch potato now that he wouldn't be programming.

By then he'd taken up daily hiking, followed by swimming and Jazzercise. As I write this, he's lost a total of 60 pounds and is back to his college weight. The type 2 diabetes breathing down his neck has disappeared, and the pins and needles of the beginning of neuropathy have faded. He now swims one mile a week and does Jazzercise, yoga, and weightlifting five times a week.

The best part of his transition is that not only did his osteoarthritis quiet down and his overall health improve, but his cognitive ability is more active than ever. He was so excited by the new science that he earned the same certificate in whole-food plant-based nutrition that I did. With this information in hand, he designed a pain management/lifestyle medicine website to support this book, https://www.BonnieLester.com.

I may have done all the cooking and made it easy for him, but he showed up with a positive attitude and a willingness to take a chance that he could feel better. The outcome exceeded both of our expectations.

My eightysomething husband is one example of how tweaking your diet can improve your health. Like I said before, there's no perfect diet for all bodies, but there are many ways to enjoy anti-inflammatory food.

In the next chapter, you'll learn about movement's magic for reducing pain. You may not be able to swim a mile like Len, but you can learn to move to feel better.

REMEMBER:

- Diet is a crucial factor in neuroplasticity.[78]

- Health-enhancing food can help reduce pain and prevent and reverse some lifestyle illnesses.

- Fiber enhances mood-elevating hormones.

- Health improvements can be achieved at any age.

---

78   "Neuroplasticity, Behavior, and Diet Intake—Rewiring the Brain for Better or Worse," The Center for Nutritional Psychology, August 23, 2021, https://www.nutritional-psychology.org/ neuroplasticity-behavior-and-dietary-intake-rewiring-the-brain-for-better-or-worse/.

CHAPTER 10

Movement's Magic for Reducing Pain

♥

"When it comes to health and well-being, regular exercise
is about as close to a magic potion as you can get."
—THÍCH NHÁT HGNH, BUDDHIST MONK, AND LILIAN CHEUNG, NUTRITIONIST

It can be daunting to consider adding movement into your life when you're in a lot of pain. When the doctor dared to tell me to exercise, I glared at him and thought, "I'll start exercising when I stop hurting."

Many people with chronic pain stop moving. All they can think about is how they want to stop hurting. They don't want to do anything to make it worse, plus their aching bodies consume them so it's hard to move. The problem is that when we don't move, our muscles weaken and our joints stiffen. Strong muscles serve as protective buffers, safeguarding our joints from wearing on each other. Toned muscles reduce tenderness and spasms, now and in the future. In addition to building a stronger body, movement also relieves stress and stimulates the release of endorphins, the body's natural pain relief neurotransmitter.

Despite knowing the benefits of exercise, since I developed CRPS, I'd been locked into a pattern that I couldn't seem to break. Every October, when the weather changed, I found myself suffering an intense flare-up that lasted until the end of March. One of the biggest contributing factors was the shift in barometric pressure.

Since you aren't meteorologists, here's a quick science lesson to explain how barometric pressure triggers flare-ups. The amount of atmospheric pressure surrounding the earth changes depending on weather and altitudes. This pressure also affects our body's joints and muscles, especially those affected by arthritis and other pain conditions. What happens is when the pressure goes low, our tissues expand, and that creates throbbing and aching in the joints.

Not everyone is affected by atmospheric pressure change, but it's a common complaint for not only people coping with chronic pain conditions but also those with epilepsy, chronic obstructive pulmonary disease, asthma, and sinus problems.

Except on rare warm winter days, the aching throughout my body knocked me off my feet for a major part of each day during winter. It became difficult to manage many of the to-dos around the house, so I got little movement into my life. The weeks clicked by as I spent most of my time in bed until I was completely out of shape. When spring finally came and my flare-up quieted, I noticed that my legs had weakened so much that it was difficult to do even the lightest of household duties, like walking into the bird room to cover my six parrot cages every evening. As soon as the weather stabilized in the spring, my suffering decreased, so I got out my cane and took brief walks in the neighborhood. By the middle of summer, I was strong enough to resume my light household duties, but I always knew I was at the mercy of the weather.

One unusual foggy July day in 2009, a year before I started walking the dogs (chapter 1), my body ached so badly my husband offered to move to a different climate to stop my weather-related suffering. Since there was no guarantee that moving to another region would solve the problem, I decided instead to dive into research to learn how I could help myself despite the ever-changing barometric pressure.

This is when I found out that it wasn't my imagination that my pain always seemed to soar when a storm was brewing. It turns out that it was due to the change in the air pressure.

Even though weather changes are inevitable, research explained that there are things we can do to feel better during dramatic shifts in air pressure. Being active and stretching and toning our muscles is a start. Also, by staying away from inflammatory foods, using heat treatments, and using NSAIDs as needed, we can reduce the discomfort caused by the barometric pressure.[79]

This information motivated me to get up off my bed and wake up my muscles by doing gentle floor stretches that included leg lifts and sitting and alternately reaching my arms above my head. It was a slow go at first, but within a couple of weeks of doing this, I felt that my muscles could take on another challenge without harming them, so I decided to add more chair exercises to strengthen my core. I also wanted to improve my balance to reduce the possibility of falling. For this I found great short chair exercise videos on YouTube. These instructional programs offer a rich source of gentle movements to strengthen and tone your body in the privacy of your home.

Many of these programs consist of a physical therapist or fitness trainer carefully explaining how to execute each gentle movement. After a few months, I engaged in "sitting cardio exercise," which required me to sit on a comfortable

---

79   "How Changes in Weather Affect Joint Pain," Cleveland Clinic, January 15, 2023, https://health.clevelandclinic.org/barometric-pressure-joint-pain/.

chair and execute movements that raised my heart rate. It also included using cans of soup for weights, which is a clever way to avoid buying hand weights.

My home-based fitness program didn't totally end the negative impact of barometric pressure changes on my body, but it did help. When my joints shouted when threatened by forecasted rain or fog, my strengthened body enabled me to not linger in bed day after day. Best of all, undertaking a daily exercise program made me feel like I was making a difference in how I felt.

If you haven't incorporated movement into your life yet, you should consider doing so. Movement improves circulation, lubricates joints, reduces swelling, and lifts your mood. Plus, it increases flexibility and strength, which helps make daily living activities easier.

Perhaps you have difficulty bending down to tie your shoes or reaching up to retrieve a can of soup from the pantry. Maybe you have discomfort reaching up and washing your hair, like I used to experience. The good news is that you can improve your range of motion to help you comfortably do these activities by consistently performing stretching exercises.[80]

I know that the last thing someone in agony wants to think about is moving their body. However, you can tailor the type of movement you choose based on your comfort level and goals. Whatever activity you choose, it's important to begin slowly.

If you decide to start an exercise program, please consult with your healthcare professional first. If you have a history of injuries, it's best to collaborate with a trained professional to work around past injuries.

When I did start moving, I wish I had known about delayed onset muscle

---

80   Becks Shepherd, "How to Increase Your Range of Motion—And Why It's Central to Your Health," Live Science, October 30, 2022, https://www.livescience.com/how-to-increase-your-range-of-motion.

soreness (DOMS), a common issue for those who are resuming physical activity after being stationary for a period of time. The onset of DOMS is due to microscopic tears occurring in the muscles.

Okay, don't freak. That sounds a lot worse than what it really is. It means that you start experiencing soreness 24 to 72 hours after your workout session. But the good news is that if you let the body do its job, those sore muscles become strong muscles.

You will know you are suffering DOMS after a workout if, in the next day or two, you start to feel muscle soreness, tenderness, and stiffness. It can be extremely uncomfortable, but it's not an indicator that there's any reason for concern.[81]

If you experience this delayed soreness, here are some self-care ways to alleviate your discomfort:

- Massage

- Hydrotherapy (spa or warm Epsom salt bath)

- Rest

- Ice pack

- Gentle stretching

- Over-the-counter topical heat rubs

It's a balancing game, and it takes discipline to show up and exercise but not overdo it. Pay close attention to the discomfort of doing the exercise. Even though weakened muscles often complain with soreness, if your exercise is causing sharp, intense pain, stop exercising. It might mean you have injured yourself. Additionally, swelling, redness, or increased warmth around a joint

---

81   Gail Olsen, "What Is Delayed Onset Muscle Soreness (DOMS) and What Can You Do About It?" Healthline, last updated November 14, 2023, https://www.healthline.com/health/doms.

or muscle immediately after exercising may be a sign of injury and should be checked out by a health-care provider.[82]

There are telltale signs to know if you're experiencing a flare-up:

- Pain in joints, muscles, and other regions of the body not related to exercise movement.

- Symptoms increase at any time, regardless of recent activity.

- Recent stress, infections, hormonal changes, poor sleep, inactivity, poor nutrition, or medication changes, which can all be flare-up triggers.

When the doctors told me to exercise, none of them explained DOMS. If they had, I wouldn't have been so resistant to starting an exercise practice. At the time, when they said "exercise," all I could think of was how much pain it would put me in and how much worse my condition would get; an explanation would have given me peace that my exercise wasn't flaring my pain condition but had a "normal" explanation. So, I tossed aside the doctors' suggestion, thinking movement was a priority for weight management and cardiovascular health, as opposed to pain management.

As you get moving, plan to wear comfortable clothes that don't constrict your range of movement. Also be aware that well-fitting shoes matter. They need to provide comfort, stability, and support to prevent injuries.

Some foot conditions work better with shoe inserts. These inserts can:

- Improve posture

- Reduce muscle fatigue

- Improve heel cushioning

---

82   Scott Harris, "How to Know if You've Injured Yourself during a Workout," Blissmark, August 22, 2021, http://www.blissmark.com/self/workout-injury/.

- Provide arch support

- Ease back, knee, and hip pain

- Provide shock absorption

If you choose to start your exercise in a swimming pool, inexpensive shoes manufactured for usage in the water can help you feel steady in the water and reduce the chance of getting foot fungus.

The following types of exercise are low impact and won't put pressure on your joints:

- Walking
- Chair or bed exercises
- Breathing exercises
- Water walking
- Stretching
- Yin Yoga
- Tai Chi

Important exercise tips:

- Pick an exercise you like doing and that best supports your body and your condition.

- Have a water bottle close by to avoid dehydration.

- Do warm-up stretches before any type of exercise that will increase your respiration and blood pressure (such as low-impact cardio or water walking). Warming-up stretches dilate your blood vessels to ensure your muscles receive a supply of oxygen, which helps prevent injuries.

- Cooling down afterward with light movement and stretches gives the body a gentle transition. This is especially important for older adults, who might struggle with regulating heart rate and blood pressure. Gradual slowdown prevents lightheadedness and fainting and encourages more blood flow, which aids in muscle recovery and diminishes the risk of getting DOMS.

Keeping these factors in mind, the guiding principle when choosing an exercise program is to select one that you enjoy doing and that supports your body and current condition. This may involve doing a variety of exercises to avoid overdoing it. Look for a low-impact exercise that doesn't put much pressure on your joints, such as stretching, walking, low-impact aerobics, Tai Chi, or Yin Yoga.

When figuring out what you want to do, think about whether you'd enjoy a social connection. If so, consider joining a group-based exercise program. City recreation departments and senior centers sponsor affordable classes for all fitness levels. Many of my clients find that working out with others is a wonderful distraction from complaining tender muscles.

Case Study: Coronary Artery Disease (CAD)

This client came to me in the most unusual way. I'd just finished completing a Walk with the Chaplain session with another client, and a thunderstorm was about to hit.

Coronary Artery Disease

CAD is a common heart condition that can be influenced by genetic factors. Although genetics can predispose you to developing CAD, poor lifestyle choices pave the way to developing it. An unhealthy eating pattern, lack of exercise, and smoking increase the risk of a buildup of cholesterol deposits in the arteries. These deposits narrow the arteries. That means that the major blood vessels are getting clogged up, making it difficult for blood carrying oxygen and nutrients to get to the heart muscle. The blocked blood flow ultimately leads to heart attacks.

Men are at greater risk of developing CAD than women are, especially if there's a family history of the disease.

Symptoms

- Chest pain (angina)

- Fatigue

- Shortness of breath

Risk Factors

- Diabetes
- Stress

- Hypertension
- Smoking

- Sedentary lifestyle

Diagnosis

- Electrocardiogram (ECG)

- Echocardiogram

- Exercise stress test

- Nuclear stress test

- Heart CT scan

- Cardiac catheterization and angiogram

Treatments

- **Angioplasty:** A minimally invasive procedure that improves blood flow in the arteries by widening narrowed or obstructed arteries. In this procedure, a catheter is inserted and then a balloon is used to create more space for the blood to circulate.

- **Stent:** A metal or plastic tube inserted to keep the artery opened and prevent it from narrowing again.

- **Coronary artery bypass graft (CABG):** Grafting healthy veins above and below the blocked artery, creating a new route for the blood to flow to bypass the narrowed or blocked coronary arteries.[83]

- **Lifestyle changes:** These might include improved diet, exercise, and stress management.[84]

On a late October afternoon, I had just completed a two-mile Walk with the Chaplain session around the football field at a local high school. I said goodbye to my client and noticed dark, threatening clouds rolling in. I hate driving in rainstorms and was hoping to make it home before the storm hit.

A tall, stocky man wearing a sweatshirt emblazoned with the school's mascot under the word "coach" approached me.

"My friend told me you help people with health problems," he said in a slight Southern drawl.

I stopped walking, noting a cigar in his fingers. I've always been extra sensitive to smoke due to my environmental allergies and didn't want any of the smoke to come in my direction. I repositioned myself to be upwind to avoid any smoke.

"I do."

83   "What Is Coronary Artery Bypass Grafting?" National Heart, Lung, and Blood Institute, March 13, 2024, https://www.nhlbi.nih.gov/health/coronary-artery-bypass-grafting.
84   "Coronary Artery Disease," Mayo Clinic, May 25, 2022, https://www.mayoclinic.org/diseases-conditions/coronary-artery-disease/symptoms-causes/syc-20350613.

He reached into his pocket and pulled out a frayed advertisement promoting our regional HMO's lifestyle medicine program. "My doc told me I should attend the classes, but I'm too busy and besides that, I don't want to be a student."

The storm clouds grew darker. "How long ago did your doctor refer you to this program?"

His eyes shifted from me as his head lowered. "Well, um, sometime last year, after I recovered from my quadruple bypass surgery."

This man was a ticking time bomb.

Trying to maintain my professional manner, I asked, "How's your recovery going?"

"Recently I had pain in my chest area, so my cardiologist ran me through tests and scans like a lab rat. I can't believe I have any blood left after all the vials they filled. Don't even get me started about the X-rays—I should be glowing."

The clouds darkened. "What did the tests show?"

"My heart's okay, but my brain's stuck in a pain pattern it created before my surgery. The doc said this program would teach me to feel better and help me avoid further cardiac surgery."

I took a step toward my car to signal I wanted to keep this conversation short. "That sounds like a great motivation to get started with the program."

"Here's the thing, my friend's wife told my wife that you used to meet with her husband, and she said you had him create paper clip chains to motivate him to eat better and exercise more. Can you do something like that for me?"

It was rare for a man to be the one who reached out concerning a health issue. It was a big deal.

"What area of the South are you from?" I asked due to his Southern drawl.

A wide grin appeared. "I'm from Marietta, Georgia. I moved to California after I graduated from Georgia Tech in 1998."

He was younger than I thought. His wrinkles and gray hair gave him the appearance of someone closer to retirement.

"I thought I recognized a Georgia accent."

"My wife got a great job offer in her computer field," he said, nodding, "so we left the humidity. I don't miss the humidity, but I sure do miss the sweet tea."

That was the opening I was looking for. The tea he was referring to is known for its cloying sweetness resulting from the high ratio of sugar to tea.

"If we work together, you're going to learn that you shouldn't be drinking sweet tea. Do you think you can handle me suggesting ways to improve your diet and add exercise into your schedule and you'll try them out?"

He shoved his hands deep into his jacket as a light wind danced between us. "Well, I can't find any authentic sweet tea around here, so that doesn't bother me. I hope you don't think I'm going to give up my favorite Southern dishes, though."

"Actually, I'm going to suggest ways you can make your favorite foods healthier."

His forehead crinkled at the thought.

If he didn't do something soon, he was going to be in real trouble.

"Let's make a deal to meet weekly for two months," I offered. "We'll discuss the healthier behaviors you need to incorporate into your life, but your part of the deal is that you *will* be doing homework, and you won't be bringing a cigar on those walks."

He looked over at his hand and dropped the cigar to the ground and stomped it out. "That's fair," he said, looking at me sheepishly. "I switched from my cigarettes to cigars, but I only smoke it for about ten minutes every couple of hours, and then I just chew on it like my old college football coach used to."

The sky had opened up and begun to sprinkle.

"Jot down the time of day and the situations that are going on when you reach for your cigar," I said, jingling my keys in my hand.

"'Kay."

"Also make a note every time you eat at a restaurant or at a fast-food place."

"Will do," he called out, running for his car.

I drove home through the drizzle that night glancing at the threatening sky and thinking about how much the coach was a potential heart attack waiting to happen. Though I heard thunder in the distance, I pulled into my driveway just as lightning streaked across the sky and rain began furiously pounding on the roof of my car.

The following week, the coach greeted me, waving his first assignment.

I took it from him and instantly spotted patterns. "Looks like you smoke and chew your cigar during tense situations."

"Yeah."

"Is it to relax?"

"Yeah."

"You know, the late Jerry Tarkanian, University of Nevada, Las Vegas's basketball coach, used to chew on a towel during games. It was an unusual but healthy way to deal with stress, but I don't expect you to chew on a towel. How about substituting sugarless gum for your cigar so you can chew away when things get tense?"

He glared at me.

"No further damage to your heart."

His shoulders slumped. "Fine, I'll buy sugarless gum on the way home."

"Great," I said with a broad smile. "Now let's talk about these frequent fast-food meals for workday lunches. These meals are high in sodium and fat."

"And expensive," he added. "Have you seen the price of hamburgers lately?"

"You'd improve your health and wallet by bringing lunch from home."

A frown appeared.

"We're talking about improving the quality of your food—we're not talking about dieting."

"Yeah, but what am I supposed to eat?"

"Fresh vegetables, fruits, potatoes, legumes, and grains will not only help your heart, improve your thinking, and elevate your moods, but they'll also work like a fountain of youth and take years off your body."

"Fine," he grumbled.

The coach and I managed to squeeze in weekly walks even as the football season ramped up. During our walks, I learned he and his wife were open to incorporating healthier food into their family's lifestyle.

I sent him home with a collection of easy heart-healthy plant-based recipes along with a list of helpful links to YouTube cooking shows.

I suggested the family watch my old reliable *Game Changers*, the documentary that got my husband on board. The documentary helped the coach's family to focus on cutting down on fast-food meals and motivated them to pack lunches for work and school.

A month later, the coach's team was on a winning streak, and the tension was rising as they faced the region's top-ranked school. He flew through his sugar-free gum, chewing one stick after another, chomping it like a meat grinder—grinding it to bits.

Next step: a new stress release.

"I know you're out on the field every day," I asked offhandedly, "but do you get any other exercise besides blowing your whistle?"

He gave me a sly smile. "Last year, while I was recovering from my surgery, I walked on my wife's treadmill. Does that count?

I shook my head. "Does the treadmill still work?"

He breathed deeply before saying, "It makes a perfect clothes rack."

"Your arteries require an investment in their health, not only by eating healthier, but by getting your blood circulating." I cleared my throat. "That means exercising every day."

He smirked.

"Your team will be impressed to see their coach looking fit."

The coach's team didn't make it to the championships that season, but the players did get to see their coach morph into a thinner, younger model than his former cigar-chewing self. Not only did his new behaviors ensure he'd be around for the next season, but the players also had the opportunity to see him jogging around the track.

My experience with the coach provided me with the ability to not only help him but also to influence his family to adopt healthy heart behaviors.

Just like the coach had to learn to be more responsible for his health, we all have the same responsibility to our overall health. Even though living with your current condition is difficult, working through lifestyle medicine's pillars will help you feel better by achieving a healthier physical and emotional state of being.

In the next chapter, you'll learn how damaging substances can increase your pain and prevent you from obtaining effective treatment. You'll learn strategies to eliminate them and start feeling better.

REMEMBER:

- Weather can increase pain, but movement can decrease its impact on your body.

- There are many low-impact exercise options to get moving and conditioning your body.

- Pacing yourself and self-awareness will help you successfully incorporate movement into your life.

- Though your muscles may groan when you start moving, you can use self-care strategies to calm them down.

CHAPTER 11

Avoiding Substances That Can Amplify Your Pain

♥

"What is addiction really? It is a sign, a signal, a symptom of distress.
It is a language that tells us about a plight that must be understood."

—ALICE MILLER, PSYCHOLOGIST

Whether it's a physical or an emotional state, no one wants to hurt. This primal desire to end suffering often finds chronic pain warriors reaching for substances to escape their agony. These substances may include nicotine, alcohol, drugs, and sugar. These things share the ability to alter your brain's chemicals and affect your perception of pain.

For the purposes of this book, rather than providing chapter and verse about the evils of these substances, we'll be focusing on how they not only cause additional health challenges but can also be an obstacle for obtaining effective treatment to diminish your pain.

Risky Substances

The Real Dangers of Smoking

It may surprise you that way back in the early to mid-1850s, people already believed cigarettes could damage your health and referred to them as "coffin nails."[85] No matter the reason someone starts smoking cigarettes, they stay with it because they are addicted. The nicotine in cigarettes triggers the brain to release dopamine, the feel-good chemical that relaxes people. The problem is that nicotine also impairs the delivery of oxygen-rich blood to the bones and tissues and hardens the arteries. There are also carcinogenic chemical compounds in it.

Smoking has been found to affect the following lifestyle diseases as well as other chronic health conditions:

- Arthritis

- Asthma

- Coronary heart disease

- Diabetes[86]

- Fibromyalgia

- High blood pressure and high cholesterol

- Lung cancer

- Chronic obstructive pulmonary disease (COPD)

- Osteoporosis

---

85   John Adler, "Coffin Nails: The Tobacco Controversy in the 19th Century," *Harp Week,* 1998–2000, https://tobacco.harpweek.com.

86   Nicotine further aggravates circulatory issues of diabetes, which can result in neuropathy, heart and kidney disease, and retinopathy.

Smoking also impairs the immune system and increases the risk of infection. Chronic pain smokers are considered poor candidates for implantable pain management devices like spinal cord stimulators. These devices deliver electrical currents along the spine to block irritating messages and are highly effective in managing migraines and other neurological conditions.

If you are looking to stop smoking, talk to your doctor about getting support through a smoking cessation group program where you will learn strategies to stick to a plan. Your doctor can also suggest nicotine replacement therapies (NRTs), like patches, gum, or nasal spray, that provide controlled doses of nicotine to reduce withdrawal symptoms as you wean yourself off nicotine. You can also try hypnotherapy, which has an effective track record.

Vaping Isn't Escaping the Coffin Nail Effect

A current popular trend involves people ditching smoking cigarettes to take up vaping. Vaping involves using an electronic device (e-cigarette) that heats nicotine with flavorings and other chemicals. Despite its name, vaping doesn't produce a pure water vapor for you to breathe. It actually creates a mist that contains addictive nicotine, propylene glycol, glycerin, and other chemicals that have been linked to cancer!

These substances are delivered as tiny particles that can permeate deep into your lungs and potentially cause permanent lung damage. What's even more crazy is that vaping can expose you to a higher level of certain toxic chemicals than traditional smoking does.[87]

Vaping can cause short-term and long-term effects.

---

87 "What Are Vaping Devices?" *National Institute on Drug Abuse*, January 8, 2020, https://nida.nih.gov/publications/drugfacts/vaping-devices-electronic-cigarettes.

Short-Term Effects

- Dry and irritated mouth and throat

- Coughing

- Eye irritation

- Headaches

- Nausea

- Shortness of breath

Long-Term Effects

- E-cigarette or vaping product use-associated lung injury (EVALI): A serious lung condition involving widespread lung damage that results in coughing, shortness of breath, and chest pain

- Asthma (or worsening of existing asthma)

- Lung scarring

- Gum disease

- Cancer

- Addiction to nicotine

- Organ damage: Vaping impacts brain development, raises blood pressure, and narrows arteries

- Leads to cigarette smoking

- Secondhand exposure: Exposes bystanders to nicotine and other chemicals

- Explosions: Batteries used in vaping devices can explode and cause burns and other serious injuries

Currently authorities are looking toward legislation to reduce the selling of e-cigarettes to minors.[88]

Drinking the Pain Away

Alcohol is another popular substance that people reach for when they want to feel better. It brings short-term relief but creates long-term consequences. Recent studies from the National Institute on Alcohol Abuse and Alcoholism suggest that around one in four adults who experience chronic pain self-medicate with alcohol.[89]

When it comes to using alcohol as a treatment for muscle spasms and other agonizing conditions, there's a problematic issue at play: the brain builds up tolerance. Our body and our brain become used to the effects of alcohol. This means we have to drink more to achieve the same amount of relief we once experienced. This opens up the danger of developing alcohol addiction.

Often people will combine alcohol with acetaminophen (Tylenol), aspirin, and opioids. Mixing alcohol with acetaminophen can lead to acute liver failure. Combining alcohol and aspirin increases the risk of gastric bleeding. Perhaps the most lethal combination is combining alcohol with opioids, which can lead to increased sedation and subsequent death due to the suppression of respiration.

The short-term relief alcohol initially provides is outweighed by the hazard it poses to the body and the considerable risk of sudden death. If you're using alcohol to manage your physical or emotional distress, consult with your physi-

---

88   Eunice Park-Lee et al., "Notes from the Field: E-Cigarette Use Among Middle and High School Students—National Youth Tobacco Survey, United States, 2021," *MMWR Morbidity and Mortality Weekly Report* 70 (2021), 1387–89, http://dx.doi.org/10.15585/mmwr.mm7039a4.

89   "The Complex Relationship Between Alcohol and Pain," National Institute on Alcohol Abuse and Alcoholism, September 27, 2019, https://niaaa.scienceblog.com/231/the-complex-relationship-between-alcohol-and-pain/.

cian to discuss treatment options. There are many low- to no-cost community resources, such as Alcoholics Anonymous (AA) and other support groups, that provide a safe place for support. Online support is also available.[90]

Unmask the Sweet Deception of Sugar and Its Hope for Healing

Sugar is everywhere. It's found in all foods that contain carbohydrates, including fruits, vegetables, dairy, and grains. This is actually a good thing. Those whole foods that contain natural sugar provide your body with a steady supply of energy.

But we also have to be aware of natural sugar's counterpart: refined sugar. Refined sugar morphs from its natural origins by going through a wild extraction process manufacturers use to intensify its flavor and extend its shelf life. High-fructose corn syrup (HFCS) and table sugar have undergone this transformation.

This supercharged sweetener has its original antioxidants and fiber stripped from it in the refining process. Its new form is inflammatory to the body and can cause joint pain and damage the blood vessels. It can cause a rapid spike in blood sugar and insulin levels that leads to a "sugar crash" (sluggishness and fatigue).

Foods that have HFCS can cause you to become resistant to leptin, the hormone that notifies your body when to eat and when to stop. This may explain the link between refined sugar and obesity. Seventy-four percent of

---

90 Jamie Becker, "The Link Between Alcohol Use and Chronic Pain," Laborers' Health and Safety Fund of North America, February 2021, https://www.lhsfna.org/the-link-between-alcohol-use-and-chronic-pain/; "Using Alcohol to Relieve Your Pain: What Are the Risks?" National Institute on Alcohol Abuse and Alcoholism, last updated May 2021, https://www.niaaa.nih.gov/publications/brochures-and-fact-sheets/using-alcohol-to-relieve-your-pain.

packaged foods have refined sugar.[91]

Here are some of those products:

- Soft drinks

- Cereals

- Yogurt

- Candy

- Cake

- Cookies

- Most processed foods, such as soups and cured meats

Excess sugar consumption can lead to:

- Obesity
- Heart disease
- Type 2 diabetes
- Hypertension
- Fatty liver disease

- Acne
- Dental decay
- Cancer
- Depression
- Cognitive problems[92]

Paying attention to labels is important to monitor your intake of sugar.

Here are other types of unhealthy sugars to look out for:

- Brown sugar

---

91   "Hidden in Plain Sight," SugarScience, accessed February 21, 2024, https://sugarscience.ucsf.edu/hidden-in-plain-sight/.

92   "The Sweet Danger of Sugar," Harvard Health Publishing, January 6, 2022, https://www.health.harvard.edu/heart-health/the-sweet-danger-of-sugar.

- Corn sweetener

- Corn syrup

- Fruit juice concentrates

- High-fructose corn syrup

- Honey

- Invert sugar

- Malt sugar

- Molasses

- Syrup sugar molecules ending in "-ose" (dextrose, fructose, glucose, lactose, maltose, sucrose)[93]

According to the National Cancer Institute, an adult male eating the standard American diet consumes an average of 24 teaspoons of added sugar per day.[94] That might not sound so bad at face value—after all, teaspoons are small— but the American Heart Association suggests that men shouldn't consume more than nine teaspoons a day (36 grams or 150 calories). Women shouldn't consume more than six teaspoons a day (25 grams or 100 calories). To put this into perspective, a 12-ounce can of soda has eight teaspoons (32 grams) of added sugar, almost a man's total sugar quota for the day and well over a woman's quota.[95]

---

93   "The Sweet Danger of Sugar."
94   "The Sweet Danger of Sugar."
95   "The Sweet Danger of Sugar."

Case Study: Complex Regional Pain Syndrome—Chaplain Bonnie Comes Clean (Yep, That's Me)

I was once a 33-year-old mom minding her own business when, through the irresponsible actions of a drunk driver, I was dragged kicking and screaming into the land of complex regional pain syndrome.

Complex Regional Pain Syndrome

Complex regional pain syndrome (CRPS) is a broad term describing prolonged and excessive inflammation and pain that follows an injury, stroke, surgery, or heart attack. The pain that develops is out of proportion to the initial severity of the injury. After living with CRPS for over three decades, I can attest to the fact that the agony I've endured was out of proportion to the injury I experienced in January 1986.

Symptoms

- Continuous burning or throbbing in the arm, leg, hand, or foot

- Sensitivity to cold or touch

- Swelling in the pain area

- Changes in skin color from white and blotchy to blue or red

- Changes in skin texture that include becoming thin, tender, or shiny

- Changes in nail and hair growth

- Joint swelling and stiffness

- Muscle spasms, tremors, and wasting of muscle mass

- Inability to move the afflicted body part

- Sweating[96]

Risk Factors

- Forceful trauma to an arm or leg

- Crushing injury or fracture

- Other traumas, such as surgery, heart attacks, and infections

Diagnosis

- Physical examination

- Nerve conduction studies

- Diagnostic imaging

- Bone scans

- Sweat production test: Warming the limbs to see if there's a discrepancy in how each limb sweats

Treatments

- Opioids

- Antidepressants

- Anticonvulsants

- Corticosteroids

- Bone-loss medications

- Sympathetic nerve-blocking medications

- Intravenous ketamine

---

96   "Complex Regional Pain Syndrome (page 1)," Mayo Clinic, accessed March 12, 2024, https://www.mayoclinic.org/diseases-conditions/crps-complex-regional-pain-syndrome/symptoms-causes/syc-20371151.

- Medications to lower blood pressure (these can sometimes help control the pain)

- Intrathecal drug pumps (medication pumped into the spinal cord fluid to relieve pain)

- Spinal cord stimulator

- Topical analgesics

- Heat therapy

- Physical and occupational therapy

- Acupuncture

- TENS unit

- Biofeedback[97]

- Neuroplasticity exercises to retrain the brain using mirror therapy or a neuro-wellness app

- Massage

- Mindfulness and cognitive behavioral therapy[98]

"Everyone has a drug of choice. Mine is smoking a pipe—what's yours?" a public health professor challenged us in our Drugs in Society class.

"Coffee," someone in the back of the room called out.

Others immediately agreed with coffee—the good old American addiction.

---

97   "Complex Regional Pain Syndrome (page 2)," Mayo Clinic, accessed March 12, 2024, https://www.mayoclinic.org/diseases-conditions/crps-complex-regional-pain-syndrome/diagnosis-treatment/drc-20371156.

98   Elena Juris, *Positive Options for Complex Regional Pain Syndrome (CRPS)* (Nashville, TN: Turner Publishing Company, 2014).

"Cigarettes," someone else said in a softer voice, clearly not as proud as the coffee drinker.

"Red wine" came from the middle.

There were a lot of nods to that one.

Others copped to the fact they couldn't say no to Kentucky Fried Chicken.

I shared none of those offered. Mine was refined sugar. It was cheap, accessible, and I always felt better after eating it. Though I tried to avoid it, when I was in the middle of menopause in 2008, it became my best friend.

My menopausal symptoms were at their peak at night, and combined with my CRPS symptoms, they made me feel like I was drowning in an ocean of hot flashes. The flashes intensified my usual burning and spasming in my neck and back. I'd reach for fat-free sweet meringues for a shot of energy and a moment of respite.

Then my tastes expanded to European dark chocolate–dipped pretzels. After all, chocolate stimulates dopamine and is good for you, right?

My husband kept a cabinet stocked with canisters of meringues and bags of my special pretzels. Then suddenly, I got my first cavity in years. Next, my cardiovascular system weighed in when my triglycerides soared. I definitely didn't need a mouthful of cavities and high triglycerides in addition to my neurological condition.

The fact was that even though meringues and pretzels were the only refined sugar treats I ate, those dear old friends hurt me and had to go. My throat choked up when I delivered my bounty of sweet treats to my neighbor.

A surprising thing happened. After enduring the sugar withdrawal, which was very real, I found that within two weeks, my body didn't ache as much.

Before we go into why, let's talk about the dear old withdrawal symptoms:

- Craving sweet foods

- Lack of energy

- Headaches

- Nausea

- Bloating

- Irritability or anxiety

- Depression or feeling down

- Stomach cramps

These symptoms are usually mild and temporary and subside as the body adjusts to lower sugar intake. Some people find the roughest part of sugar withdrawal is the psychological impact. Sugar triggers the release of endorphins, which are our body's natural opioids. For a lot of us, that means that when we are feeling stressed, tired, or uncomfortable, getting a hit of sugar will calm us. Unfortunately, so far, I haven't experienced vegetables having quite the same effect.

I have clients claim that the hardest part of sugar withdrawal is feeling unsatisfied, like they're missing something and not quite sure what it is. More healthy food will not give them that immediate high.

What's happened is our brains have become dependent on the sugar for its bump. We associate positive emotion with sugar. It's scary to think about cutting out refined sugar. When we do avoid it, in effect, we're temporarily knocking out the brain's reward system.

For me, tapering off refined sugar was easier than tapering off opioids. I slowly reduced my sugar intake instead of doing it cold turkey. Thankfully, my detox symptoms were only a slight headache for a day or two and a longing for a sugar high, which I soothed by enjoying oven-caramelized roasted yams.

I also made sure to up my game to stimulate my happy chemicals. My dog walking, gardening, and chatting with friends lifted my spirits as I said goodbye to my sugar treats. I also placed relaxation tapes on my nightstand to use in the middle of the night instead of grabbing for a hit of refined sugar.

Next, I addressed my dental health by instituting a new dental cleaning regime. I bought a Waterpik to use along with my electric brush and flossing thread. I soon received glowing reports from my dental hygienist.

My refined sugar detox occurred 15 years ago and since then, my favorite sweet treats that make me smile but protect my health include a bowl of fruit doused in huckleberry balsamic vinegar and a simple baked apple sprinkled with cinnamon.

As far as my improvement from CRPS, the past 10 chapters have already chronicled the helpful strategies I used to feel much better.

You can see from my battle with refined sugar that we can further damage our health by searching for relief in the wrong places. Once you identify the damaging substances in your life, you can also take steps to eliminate them and their impact on your condition.

In the next chapter, we're going to slay our negative thoughts and emotions that elevate our stress response and increase our suffering.

REMEMBER:

- Some substances not only damage your health but can prevent you from getting effective pain management treatment.

- Vaping is worse than smoking.

- It's deadly to combine alcohol with opioids.

- Some substances can increase your pain.

- Refined sugar is not your friend.

CHAPTER 12

Bounce Back
Against All Odds

♥

"The greatest weapon against stress is our ability to choose one thought over another."

—ATTRIBUTED TO WILLIAM JAMES, PSYCHOLOGIST AND PHILOSOPHER

"Bonnie, I know you have a rare pain condition," my totally fit 33-year-old physical therapist said. She pressed on a deep trigger point that throbbed in my left shoulder blade. "The truth is that everyone's at risk of having their suffering increased by stress."

It took a moment for the significance of what she was saying to land. Slowly, my mind opened to how universal pain was in the human condition and the negative consequences that could result from that. There was comfort and a sadness that came from knowing that I wasn't unique, nor alone, with my experience.

When she mentioned that stress was making my pain worse, it was clear that if I wanted to feel better, I needed to figure out how to have less of it. I was no longer down on myself because I had implemented mindfulness and cognitive behavioral strategies (chapter 7), but I still felt the weight of life's pressures bearing down on me. It was time to research lifestyle medicine's fourth pillar to figure out how to improve my response.

♥

"It's not stress that kills us; it's our reaction to it."
—Attributed to Hans Selye

Stress is a hot topic that sweeps through social media like an angry storm. Let's face it: none of us can duck and hide from stress. Work pressures, family conflicts, the constant strain of children, gridlock traffic, health challenges, finances, grieving personal loss, or even moving—all these things can do a number on us.

When stress hits, our bodies kick into fight or flight. That's why stress is a survival thing. Our heroic brains immediately release hormones, gearing us up to either battle the pending danger or hightail it to safety. Stress is our own built-in superhero response to save ourselves.

But here's the kicker: prolonged exposure to stress is a buzzkill for our mental health and overall well-being. So, it's high time we figure out creative ways to tackle it head-on and give it a one-two punch.

To be successful doing this, we need to know the secrets of taming stress. The first secret is to understand that, whether we're putting too much pressure on ourselves or having pressure placed on us by others (maybe we're trying to get our kids out the door to catch the bus, or we're trying to meet a tight deadline at work), our bodies go through the same physiological response. First the muscles tense, then blood pressure and respiration increase to give us the oomph to deal with a challenge. Here's the catch: if this heightened response is left on too long, it damages our health.

Back in 1936, Hans Selye, a Hungarian-born researcher, coined the term "stress" to label the physical, mental, and emotional influences that stimulate the release of hormones and chemicals. He divided these stressors into good stress (eustress) and bad stress (distress).[99]

Eustress, the good kind of stress, motivates you and occurs for a limited period. It focuses your energy, creates a sense of excitement, and improves your performance. Examples of eustress include receiving a job promotion, learning a new skill, taking a relaxing vacation, participating in sports competitions, and planning a party. This type of stress, if handled right, doesn't take a toll on your body and is considered beneficial for motivation, performance, and well-being.

Too much of the bad kind of stress, distress, can mess us up. It leads to what we call "stress overload." It's like your body's regulation system goes on strike, screaming, "Enough already." When this happens, the brain's alert system sticks in high gear like the Energizer Bunny, never stopping. This wears your body and mind down. If you're dealing with chronic pain, you're the lucky winner to have pain and overload as your constant companions.

But we do have an ace in the hole to fight this fierce invasion of your body's heightened response. It's called "fun." Yes, you heard me; by indulging in enjoyable activities and remembering the good times, you're giving that nasty stress a good old-fashioned beatdown.

For success in this undertaking, we need to identify what is contributing to the attack so we can defend ourselves with additional tools to minimize its impact.

---

99   Beth Frates et al., *Lifestyle Medicine Handbook: An Introduction to the Power of Healthy Habits* (Monterey, CA: Healthy Learning, 2021).

Types of Factors That Can Cause a Negative Overload

External Factors

- Abuse
- Chemical toxins
- Cold weather
- Domestic violence
- Environmental factors
- Financial problems
- Hot weather
- Mold
- Pandemic
- Traffic
- Work issues or unemployment

Internal Factors

- Allergies
- Excessive caffeine
- Excessive exercise
- Illness
- Injury
- Insomnia
- Obesity
- Pain
- Processed food
- Risky substances
- Sedentary lifestyle

Psychological Factors

- Anxiety
- Chemical imbalances
- Depression
- Fear
- Pessimism
- Unrealistic expectations

Symptoms can include:

- Acne
- Anxiety
- Blurred vision
- Clenched jaw
- Compromised immune system
- Constipation
- Dilated eyes
- Difficulty concentrating
- Decreased sex drive
- Depression
- Dry mouth
- Emotional issues
- Eye tics
- Feeling dizzy and jittery due to the extra oxygen in the blood stream
- Headaches
- Increased sensitivity to sounds
- Insomnia
- Muscle spasms
- Pain in the diaphragm from increased respiration
- Racing heart
- Rashes and itching
- Suicide

These physical and emotional symptoms are obvious. What might not be so obvious is that these external forces can act as our own personal kryptonite, messing with all our bodies' systems.

Here are some of the ways stress affects the body:

- **Circulatory system (blood circulation):** When people are stuck in fight-or-flight mode for a protracted period of time, the heart rate and blood pressure elevate. This increases the risk of stroke and heart attack.

- **Endocrine system (hormone secretions):** Excessive stress disrupts regulating growth hormones, metabolism, and reproduction systems.

This leads to weight gain or difficulty losing weight. It can also create problems in the menstrual cycle and cause fertility issues.

- **Gastrointestinal system (digestion):** Stress elevates stomach acid, which harms the stomach. It can also lead to indigestion and changes in bowel habits, leading to diarrhea or constipation.

- **Immune system:** When stress is high, it suppresses the immune system's production of virus-killing cells. This increases the risk of getting sick and can also make chronic conditions worse.

- **Integumentary system (body's outer skin):** The increased pressure can make the skin more sensitive and reactive. That can lead to hives or other skin conditions. Healing is also slowed, making it take longer for bruises and other skin wounds to heal.

- **Muscular system (movement):** Prolonged strain causes the muscles to become chronically tense. This makes a person more likely to experience headaches, migraines, and related pain in the muscles as well as alignment issues.

- **Nervous system (coordination of actions and senses):** Stress produces changes in the structure of the brain and may impact memory, decision-making, and emotional regulation.

- **Renal/urinary system (excretion):** Stress raises our blood pressure, which, in turn, hammers our body's waste elimination process. It damages the kidneys, making it harder for our toxins to be filtered out. Plus, it triggers the bladder to tighten, making us run to the bathroom more often.

- **Reproductive system (sexual reproduction):** Chronic stress puts a halt to the production of sperm in men. In women, it can stop the menstrual cycle. Women, before you start thinking that this is a good thing, having no cycle reduces the level of estrogen, which is necessary for maintaining bone health and staying wrinkle-free.

Over time, the loss of bone density increases the risk of osteoporosis.

- **Respiratory system (breathing):** When we worry, our breathing becomes more rapid and shallow. This means less oxygen reaches our bloodstream. Breathing at such a pace can lead to dizziness, tingling sensations in our hands and feet, and chest tightness. Oftentimes this leads to hyperventilation or panic attacks. If you already have respiratory issues, things will worsen.

- **Skeletal system:** Long-term exposure leads to decline in bone density, which in turn raises the risk of fractures and osteoporosis.

As you can see, all our bodies' biological systems take a hit from long-lasting stress. For those who already struggle with chronic pain, the damage it produces is an additional blow that we are ill-equipped to handle.

After doing a deep dive into how badly stress affected my body, I immersed myself in figuring out when it was making my condition worse. I stewed on the times when I felt the most wigged out. It didn't take long to figure out that it was when I doubted how I handled a situation. I'd dwell on the what-ifs or if-onlies, followed up by gigantic heaps of "I can't believe he said that." Every time those dang thoughts popped up, my stomach tightened like it had suffered a hard punch.

As a countertactic, I decided to tame the wild stallion of negative thoughts and give my stomach a break. To do this, I needed to not become so upset by things happening in my life. When someone cut in line at the store, I told myself, "Stay calm; don't let it bug you." But I still found myself grinding my teeth and glaring at the line cutter.

When someone almost hit me with their car, anger pounded through me, letting the stress win again.

After this went on for a couple of weeks, I decided I had to better arm myself. The best place to find instructions for this was my mindfulness and CBT books. I dove deep into my resources and found strategies like deep breathing, visualization, and grounding exercises based on the five senses. There was a lot of evidence in science research that these methods would provide a good defense.[100]

I was armed for war when, a few days later, the physician assistant from my doctor's office called. I was driving on the highway. I pulled over to the shoulder of the road to hear the update about my health.

"Your results came in from the scan, and they're inconclusive," she said with her usual even-keeled voice.

My heart pounded. I took a deep, cleansing breath. "Stay calm," I told myself as I exhaled, and then "Stay focused." I concentrated on the physician assistant's words as she explained my options to nail down a diagnosis.

"It's up to you to decide if you want to have another type of scan or schedule a biopsy."

She hung up, and cars whizzed by. I breathed in for five counts and let the air out for seven, over and over again. As my heart settled, I straightened my shoulders. My rib cage and diaphragm expanded more with each deep breath. I closed my eyes and exhaled, visualizing the tension in my body evaporating.

I opened my eyes and described what was around me using the five senses.

"I see five crows on a chain-link fence."

"The sound of traffic changes whenever a truck speeds by."

---

100 J. David Creswell and Bassam Khoury, "Mindfulness Meditation: A Research-Proven Way to Reduce Stress," American Psychological Association, October 30, 2019, https://www.apa.org/topics/mindfulness/meditation.

"I smell my herbal tea in my travel cup."

"I can taste the cinnamon in my herbal tea."

"The heated car seat feels good on my back."

These exercises signaled to my alert system to down-regulate. I found myself calming enough that I was safe to drive. By the time I made it home, I had weighed out the situation and knew the right thing for me to do was to set up an appointment for another type of scan. A week later, I received an "all clear" report.

With one victory under my belt, I was ready to attack other problematic areas. I went on high alert for sneaky fight-or-flight attacks. Soon. I detected that throughout the day, I worried about being a stepmom to a teenage son and daughter, plus how to blend my college-aged son into the mix so he'd feel comfortable.

Well, all that doubting gave the attacker the competitive advantage, and it needed to be disarmed. To do that, my strategy was to allow myself 15 minutes to think about disappointments and doubts. Then, after that, it was a don't-think-about-it zone.

When the thoughts came, I spoke back to them. "Our newly blended family is an exciting opportunity for all five of us to grow and strengthen our bonds. I'm taking it one day at a time. I trust that I'll know what to do when it's time to do something. My son will be fine. He's strong and has always coped well with change."

Do you know what happened? Stress retreated, and my overall energy increased. Eventually, I talked back to my doubts so often that they stopped showing up! With them no longer hanging around, I became a lot happier.

When you practice relaxation and mindfulness exercises, your resiliency will increase, and you'll be better equipped to reduce the impact of unhealthy challenges in your life.

Below are more battle techniques that I have found to be extremely helpful.

The Power of Acknowledgment

Many of us, including myself, underestimate the power acknowledgment can have. At the heart of this practice, it requires recognizing, valuing, and voicing gratitude for the good aspects, achievements, and qualities in our lives. To make something truly an act of acknowledgment, we also are required to express appreciation for what we are honoring.

No matter how small or big something is, by appreciating and fully acknowledging it, we are shifting our mindset from negativity and lack to positivity and abundance. This cultivates a happier outlook on life. That in turn releases all the good chemicals. Our sense of well-being improves and so does our resilience.[101]

A few ways you can increase the act of acknowledgment in your life:

- Every morning, jot down three to five things you are thankful for.

- Label a jar "Good Things" and, at the end of each day, jot down the day's positive events and how they made you feel. You'll be surprised how fast your jar will be filled with "good things."

- Once a week, send a text, email, or letter or leave a comment on social media telling someone how pleased you are that they're in your life.

---

101   Madhuleena Roy Chowdhury, "Neuroscience of Gratitude and the Effects on the Brain," Positive Psychology, April 9, 2019, https://positivepsychology.com/neuroscience-of-gratitude/.

Self-Compassion: Your Precious Gemstone

Self-compassion is when a person treats themselves with as much love as they would treat other people who are dear to them. Research has shown that actively practicing self-compassion daily improves our physical health.[102] To truly show ourselves self-compassion, we have to accept our imperfections, practice forgiveness, let go when we mess up, and notice the things we have done well.

Personally, I like to practice self-compassion by starting out each day with exploring some of my past challenges and congratulating myself for successfully overcoming them. Naturally, there are times when I come up short, but instead of getting down on myself and drowning in a tidal wave of shame, I acknowledge that I'm human and that part of that means not always getting things right.

When we are kinder to ourselves, it not only boosts our mental well-being, but it also gives a charge to our physical health, including strengthening our immune system, causing our hearts to be stronger, and sometimes even extending our lifespan.[103] If those aren't enough reasons to regularly practice self-compassion, it also leads to us taking on other healthier habits since that is the loving thing to do.

---

102 Michelle Brooten-Brooks, "What Is Self-Compassion?" Verywell Health, May 23, 2022, https://www.verywellhealth.com/self-compassion-5220012.

103 Juliana Breines, "Can Being Kind to Yourself Improve Health?" Psychology Today, September 30, 2021, https://www.psychologytoday.com/us/blog/in-love-and-war/202109/can-being-kind-yourself-improve-health.

Pep Talk Yourself to Mental Toughness

Oftentimes a good old pep talk can help us climb out of the pit. Choosing the best one to give yourself depends on your personality. Pick the kind that will get you out of the dumps. One way to do this is to focus on your strengths, your skills, your wins, and why you're wanting what you're wanting. This will strengthen your resilience and reduce the tension that you might be carrying around without realizing it.

My personal favorite way to do this is to breathe in while thinking about all my strengths. Breathing exercises help me focus on the present moment, enhancing my receptiveness to the words I am telling myself.

Pep Talk Breathing Exercise

1. Breathe in for six seconds. Hold it for two seconds. Breathe out for seven seconds.

2. Visualize all the things you've done well in the past day.

3. Visualize yourself accomplishing activities you need to do today.

4. Repeat "I can do this" for five seconds.

5. Finish with a breath cycle of breathing in for six seconds, holding for two, and exhaling for seven.

Trial by Fire

A few weeks after I began implementing my calming reaction program, my refrigerator and oven stopped working. Normally, not being able to prepare my food would have sent my panic meter over the top.

This time, I immediately jumped into focused rounds of deep breathing and observing my environment while I was on hold on the phone for over an hour with our home warranty company. Finally, I was able to schedule a service person to fix both appliances.

The next day, I was dealt another challenging issue when a rodent control company stopped by to explore why a strange smell was emanating from my husband's office in our recently remodeled home. We were appalled to learn it was due to a rat's corpse stuck between the walls. The rodent had secured itself out of the reach of the company's equipment, making easy removal impossible. We had to decide whether to demolish the wall or close off the room for months and depend on Mother Nature to take its course. Not wanting to deal with further construction, we closed off the room.

When the rodent company guy collected his equipment from my backyard, he pointed out that the foundation for my art studio we were building was cracking. Long story short, the contractor had laid the foundation wrong, and I was forced to have my dream studio demolished.

With each of these events, I vigorously applied the mindfulness and relaxation exercises until my stomach had no knots and I could move forward empowered. That proved I could take that bad old stress and whittle it down in size, even in the most challenging circumstances. (Yes, I did get a full refund on the art studio).

Case Study: Chronic Postsurgical Pain

On a sunny September day at noon, I slipped under a redwood tree for its shade. I stood next to Sproul Hall, located in the heart of the University of California, Berkeley's campus. The hall had classical revival columns covered with flyers announcing upcoming concerts and lectures. I was waiting for a friend, Lena, a seismology (study of earthquakes) doctoral candidate and teaching assistant. Her passion for this topic had grown from the tales she had heard over the years about her distant relatives surviving the 1906 San Francisco earthquake.

A buzzing sea of young people hustled about, wearing the ever-popular college uniform of blue jeans. Backpacks were slung over shoulders, and most eyes were glued to phones. Four students sat on a bench signing in American Sign Language. Food trucks lined the street and filled the air with the scents of spicy falafel and barbecue ribs. My tummy rumbled, reminding me it was lunchtime, just as I spied Lena walking in my direction.

Her dark brown hair flowed down her back, and her deep blue eyes contrasted dramatically with her smooth olive skin tone. The grace she walked with and her well-defined muscles were a by-product of her love for long-distance running.

She'd often recruited me to sponsor disease fundraiser road races over the years. We were meeting because she was aware of my pain recovery experience and training, and she wanted assistance with her newfound chronic pain following foot surgery to remove a benign growth of nerve tissue from the ball of her foot. Prior to the surgery, the nerve tissue felt like she was standing on a small pebble all the time, but since the surgery, her foot had been more tender and had a constant burning sensation.

Chronic Postsurgical Pain

Chronic postsurgical pain (CPSP) is a condition that can happen after a person has surgery. Even after the body has healed and stitches are removed, the pain from the surgery continues.[104]

---

104 Erica Jacques, "What Causes Chronic Postoperative Pain?" Verywell Health, last updated November 13, 2022, https://www.verywellhealth.com/what-causes-chronic-postoperative-pain-2564559.

Symptoms
- Sharp stabbing sensation
- Throbbing
- Burning
- Numbness

Risk Factors

- Nerve damage during surgery
- Scar tissue forming during the healing process that may compress or irritate nerve endings
- Tissue damage
- Wound inflammation

Diagnosis

- Symptoms meet certain criteria, including pain that developed after a surgical procedure, pain of two to three months' duration, other causes for the pain can be excluded, and no known preexisting condition or cause

Treatments
- NSAIDs
- Tylenol
- Opioids
- Anticonvulsants
- Nerve blocks
- Ketamine
- TENS unit
- Physical therapy
- Massage
- Mindfulness-Based Cognitive Behavioral Therapy
- Lifestyle management

After Lena and I greeted each other with a warm hug, we moved to a quaint outdoor café and ordered lunch.

Once the food came, she dug into her taco salad. "Due to my darn CPSP, I'm not running road races anymore, so I have no need for a carbo load."

I looked down at my veggie burrito, mulling over this sad turn of events for my friend.

"I'm able to limp to my school classes on my worst days," she continued, "but I had to cancel participating in a brain cancer fundraiser run last month."

That let me know just how bad this condition was for her. I stewed for a moment, mulling over the best way to begin. "Are you receiving treatment at the college health center?"

"They put me on an anti-inflammatory, but that didn't stop the throbbing. The doc also suggested I wear lighter track shoes with orthotic inserts to alleviate pressure."

After swallowing my bit of burrito, I asked, "How's that working for you?"

"I found one that sorta helps."

Lena went on to explain that at her recent follow-up appointment, the doctor had suggested she use an app, Wave Health (www.wavehealth.app), to discover her pain triggers. "The app helped me discover that stress, weather changes, and certain foods are the big three in my pain life."

"Well, unless you're up for moving to another climate, let's focus on helping you avoid the foods the app identified as triggers and work on life management skills to reduce your stress."

She shook her head. "Even though the app says stress is a trigger, I'm handling everything fine. I've got a 4.0, and I'm really disciplined about my research and teaching. I'm staying on top of everything."

"That's impressive." I took a sip of Perrier, then said, "I'm curious, do you relax during the week?"

She gave me a weary smile. "Every now and then I check out Instagram. I also catch a flick on Amazon Prime…sometimes."

I replaced the cap on my bottle of carbonated mineral water and gave it a shake every time I mentioned a possible college pressure.

"Maintaining a high GPA is one shake." I shook my bottle.

"Steep college tuition, another shake."

"Waiting to hear if your grant's been funded…a real big shake."

I held my bottle up high so she could see the fizz and bubbles. "What do you think would happen if I took off the cap right now?"

"It'd explode."

"Our body needs a release valve."

She looked at my bubbling water bottle and nodded that she got what I was saying.

"Why don't we discuss simple things you can do to dial it down to help your pain?"

She raised an eyebrow. "Do you really think my pain can be lowered if I relax?"

"Do you notice your foot pain when someone asks you about your family's experience in the 1906 San Francisco earthquake?"

"You know that's my favorite subject, so I wouldn't be focusing on my foot."

"When you shift into your storytelling mode, your body relaxes, which lessens the pain. Taking time to achieve a relaxed state in your busy day will pay dividends in quieting down your discomfort."

She squinted her blue eyes as she processed.

"Since you're a science nerd, I'm going to give you a link to a site that will describe the physiological impact stress has on the body. It can even alter our memory and our ability to concentrate."

She moved her plate away from her after she finished eating. "I don't like hearing that."

"It's a problem for your entire body, but you can learn how to defuse its impact. Let's meet through Zoom next week so we can talk about how not taking time to just relax can impact your pain."

Before we parted, I called out, "I'm happy to sponsor you if you participate in the Cystic Fibrosis Foundation Walkathon I heard about on the radio today."

Lena grinned as she waved goodbye.

Dancing the waltz with chronic pain means accommodating it whenever it steps on your toes. Sometimes favorite routines and enjoyable recreational activities have to be modified temporarily. Adopting flexible goals provides adaptability to the unpredictable nature of pain. This allows individuals to make adjustments that are practical and attainable in order to enhance their well-being.[105]

The following week, I Zoomed in and got a glimpse of Lena's research-laden

---

105   Lawrence Roux, Sylvia M. Gustin, and Toby R. O. Newton-John, "To Persist or Not to Persist? The Dilemma of Goal Adjustment in Chronic Pain," *Pain* 163, no. 5 (2021), https://doi.org/10.1097/j.pain.0000000000002503.

apartment. She was in study mode—her hair was pulled back in a no-nonsense ponytail, and her black octagon-shaped wire-rimmed glasses were perched on the bridge of her nose. Towers of reports were stacked on top of a bookshelf that was crammed with textbooks. On the wall behind her, I spied her famous San Francisco earthquake photos alongside three luxurious dark green wall plants. She obviously had a green thumb.

"I still don't think I'm overwhelmed," Lena immediately declared.

"When your dissertation advisor sends you an email with remarks about your latest submission, does your stomach tighten in anticipation of her words?"

"Of course."

"How about being stuck in bumper-to-bumper traffic on your way to your parents' house for dinner?"

"Ugh, I don't know anyone who likes that."

"Are you preoccupied thinking about obtaining further funding for your fellowship position?"

She frowned. "Wouldn't you be worried if you spent all this time and money on your schooling?"

"I get you have a busy schedule and you're excelling in your field, but it seems like you're treating the pressures in your life as inconveniences that you just push through."

"Well, what else am I supposed to do?"

"I'm not suggesting that you don't deal with these items, but I'm saying that the pressure of those things is adding up and playing havoc with your health, unless you have ways to release the built-up tension these issues cause. If you counteract them with some calming time, the pain in your foot will be dialed down."

The idea of being in less pain caught her attention. She grabbed a pen to take notes.

"First thing in the morning, take time to focus on acknowledging all the good qualities and accomplishments you have going on in your life. Starting the day that way stimulates happy chemicals."

"That's simple enough." She wrote it down. "I can handle that."

"Here's another assignment that involves casting your mind in a new role— Lena's Motivator. You can use the initials LM to keep it streamlined."

"LM, huh?"

"That's right. LM is going to give you the exact type of pep talk you need to resist the negative thoughts that bombard you. LM will help build up your happy chemicals by reminding you of your strengths and wins."

She stared at me. "How's that supposed to help my foot?"

"When you stimulate happy chemicals, it triggers your body's natural ability to reduce pain."

"Got it."

"Whenever a challenge pops up, LM will remind you of all the positive things in your life."

"I'll give it a try. I can't wait to have less pain."

The next week, Lena Zoomed in from her backyard, wearing a yellow floral sundress and a floppy wide-brimmed straw hat.

"What a beautiful garden." A slight breeze caused tall pink hollyhocks to dance in the background.

"I couldn't resist sitting in the sun." She brushed her hair off her face.

"How did your new buddy LM work out for you?"

She giggled. "She's a gem and a real keeper. As soon as my feet hit the floor every morning, she reminds me that our day's mission is to keep my mood stabilizer chemicals high."

"How's your foot?"

"I only really notice when my mood is down, and then I have discomfort when I'm walking. I'm itching to get back to running," she wistfully added.

"When you do go running, how do you prepare for the long runs?"

She went into detail about her stretching routine but also how she did breathing exercises and visualization about how good she'd feel crossing the finish line.

These exercises ready the runner's mind for the challenge of running. They put the individual's mind in the zone and control the rhythm of breathing, which improves the oxygen flow to the muscles. This triggers the release of endorphins, the natural painkillers of the body.

"It's time to dust off the visualizations and breathing exercises you were doing when you prepared to do long-distance runs because they're perfect to help you relax. Rather than visualizing getting to a race finish line, visualize yourself moving comfortably throughout your day."

Lena soon became too busy to meet, and we resorted to texts. She informed me that she keeps a mason jar on her kitchen counter and fills it with positive notes. It serves as a visual cue to keep her spirits up. She learned to squeeze in her meditation and breathing exercises when her students file out after class. On weekends, I'd receive a thumbs-up emoji with a photo of her relaxing at a concert or a play. Sometimes she'd send out a screenshot of an interesting show on Netflix she was enjoying.

Her big breakthrough was obvious when she sent me an email recruiting sponsors for an upcoming breast cancer fundraising walkathon. Not only did I sign on, but I called her up to congratulate her on returning to her passion of being involved with these types of fundraisers.

Lena's CPSP still remains, but its pain volume level is low. She's on a low-dose anti-inflammatory that's helping, and she has a closet full of comfortable shoes to accommodate her foot issue. She's also become an advocate for the affordable off-the-shelf orthotics that make a difference in her comfort level.

Both Lena and I took on how we interacted with our world to calm down our pain. Using the power of acknowledgment, cutting ourselves some slack, and using pep talks made a difference in our lives, as it can in yours.

In the next chapter, you'll learn how lack of sleep negatively impacts your 11 biological systems and how to take steps today to establish a sleeping pattern so you wake up feeling refreshed.

REMEMBER:

- There's good stress and bad stress.
- Bad stress negatively impacts all 11 of our biological systems.
- Physiological changes due to stress amplify pain.
- Our body's response to stress can be managed with mind-body techniques.
- Relaxation is a key ingredient to ease pain.

CHAPTER 13

Sweet Slumber

♥

"Sleep is the best meditation."

—ATTRIBUTED TO THE 14ᵀᴴ DALAI LAMA, SPIRITUAL LEADER

"I might be winning in other areas of my health rehabilitation program, but I'm certainly failing at getting any sleep," I thought for the thousandth time.

I kicked at my sheets, fighting my way out of the tangled mess. Frustrated, I rolled over with a thump to glare at the darn clock. Midnight. I sighed. I had no signs that sleep was coming.

1 a.m. Still staring at the red numbers.

2 a.m. Getting panicked that I wouldn't get any sleep.

4 a.m. Nothing was getting better.

5 a.m. The early morning garbage pickup rumbled outside, waking up the entire neighborhood.

I shoved my feet into my slippers, frustrated that sleep had evaded me for another night. This was the way it had gone for almost three decades, and no, I wasn't getting used to it. My entire body craved sleep. But, I thought, examining the blackest circles under my eyes in my bathroom mirror, I'd figure this out.

I combed my hair and slapped on lipstick to look alive as I faced another day. This sleep challenge had spanned the length of two of my marriages. I was better at not sleeping than staying married, even though I ensured that my lack of catching zzz's didn't disturb my husbands' sleep.

Sometimes I crawled out of bed unable to stare at the clock anymore and divided my time between the guest room, office, and living room. Some nights I plunged into movie marathons, and on other nights, I read. When my son was 10, he asked, "Mom, where're you going to sleep so we can do the movie marathon together?"

But all wasn't lost. Often, my body would pass out around four and wake up to dash into the day at seven. That meant that if I was lucky, I earned three hours of sleep.

Despite my ongoing struggle with not sleeping, I stubbornly resisted taking prescription or over-the-counter sleeping pills. I lived in fear of what sleeping and diet pills could do to a person's life, as reenacted in the movie *Valley of the Dolls* I'd watched at 15.

Insomnia never loosened its grip. In fact, it became worse when we went on family vacations where I was stuck in the room with family, knowing I couldn't watch the TV into the early morning hours. In hopes of making it through the night, I packed plenty of books and a flashlight. When the iPad became available back in 2008, I used Bluetooth technology to watch documentaries to help make the time pass.

Sleeplessness isn't rare. A lot of people with chronic pain conditions earn the affliction, and so do women tiptoeing to menopause. Of course, so do those people who work at pressure-cooker jobs or students stressed about their grades. Also, let's not forget those parents who suffer sleepless nights due to winning the lottery of having colicky babies.

Years into my sleeping struggle, Dr. Redhead suggested an antidepressant (not a sleeping pill) that not only calmed nerve pain but also caused drowsiness. Instead of improving my sleep, it intensified my lack of sleep hangover and added unwanted pounds. I gave up on any type of medication recommended for sleep.

In the 1990s, the mind-body movement rippled through the country. The "whole person" approach to health and wellness hit the headlines and caused herbal shops to pop up across the country to heal bodies by using natural remedies rather than prescriptions. This trend caught my attention. I'd already had success using ginger for nausea, so using herbs to sleep sounded like a possible option. Convinced that a botanical concoction wouldn't turn out like *Valley of the Dolls*, I made my way to my own local herbal shop to find that hundreds of colorful jars filled the walls of the store. There were also bins of ginger, echinacea, and licorice root contributing to the spicy aroma filling the air.

The young herbalist with auburn hair tied in a ponytail stood at the cash register engaged in a lively conversation with a willowy silver-haired woman about how papaya enzymes aid digestion problems.

He looked in my direction. "I'll be with you in just a moment."

The customer nodded at me, then tucked her bag full of supplements into her shoulder bag and left.

When I explained my quest for sleep-inducing herbs, the herbalist's blue eyes sparkled. He reached into the cabinet behind him and handed me a white plastic bottle. "You'll sleep through the night with this."

I read the back label: "Apigenin is a natural bioactive compound to induce sleep and promote relaxation." It sounded great.

That evening, I popped the pill and waited for the much-needed sleep. I didn't drift into dreamland, though; my eyes itched and my nose got stuffy, like I had wandered through a field of wildflowers brimming with pollen.

I anxiously grabbed the pill bottle and squinted at the label. For the first time, a tiny ornate gold-scripted word came into focus: chamomile. A tight knot immediately formed in my stomach. I'm extremely allergic to chamomile. With a sense of dread, I fumbled through my medicine cabinet and, finding my allergy pills, I downed one with a huge glass of water, hoping I had taken it in time to counter a full-on allergy attack. After that, I disgustedly tossed the herbal supplement into the trash.

Flowers and plants have been used for thousands of years for healing, but just because they come from nature, that doesn't take away the powerful effect they can have on the body. FDA rules have improved their labeling, but these rules also put strong limits on what can and can't be said on the packages. Use caution and professional guidance when choosing supplements.

Things to Consider About Herbal Supplements

- Consult with professionals like herbalists, naturopathic doctors, and those acupuncturists who have training in herbal medicine.

- Select supplements that provide a toll-free telephone number, address, or website address. That contact information provides the consumer with an avenue to find out further details about the ingredients, what testing methods were used to develop the product, and possible adverse interactions with prescription medications.

- Inform your health-care professional whenever you take herbal supplements. Supplements can react with other medications and impact their potency, leading to side effects. There's also a danger of overdosing on vitamins and minerals.

- Read the labels on your supplements, even if you have to get out your magnifying glass to see the print. Hint: if the print is impossible to read on the bottle because of print size, look up the supplement bottle online and increase the font size over the ingredients picture or in the description section.

- If you're sensitive, it's best to start with a low dosage to see how your body reacts.

- Never exceed the recommended dosage unless instructed by a health professional.

- Pay attention to side effects. If you experience symptoms such as headache, nausea, dizziness, itchiness, rash, swelling, or stomach-ache, discontinue the supplement immediately.

- If you have trouble breathing, call 911 or the emergency number for your area.[106]

Given my lifelong dance with environmental allergies, playing with herbal supplements seemed like flirting with disaster. Yes, I could brave herbal teas every once in a while, but I was also the person who, after sniffing a lovely bouquet of flowers, could spiral into a sneezing fit that could last for hours. My better judgment was to steer clear of those natural concoctions to avoid a negative outcome. Not willing to give up my desire for a good night's sleep, I hit the medical books again, this time determined to find a miracle remedy.

---

106 Oladimeji Ewumi, "What Is Herbal Medicine, and What Are the Benefits?" Medical News Today, October 6, 2022, https://www.medicalnewstoday.com/articles/herbal-medicine.

The Lowdown on Sleep

The range of hours of sleep that people need to be healthy varies wildly, but to earn the title of insomnia, you have to struggle for three months in a row for at least three nights each week. I easily earned that medal. In fact, I daresay I took gold on that one.

But apparently, I wasn't the only one. The study of sleep goes back to Aristotle's time. He theorized that sleep is a time of physical renewal. He believed it was initiated by warm vapors rising from the heart during digestion.[107] Centuries later, contemporary sleep scientists found that sleep is when the total body is actively restoring itself.

Picture a skyscraper that houses businesses during the day. The elevators, lobbies, restrooms, and cafés are crowded from morning until sunset. When night arrives, the heavily trafficked common areas need to be cleaned and polished. That's what our body does while we sleep. Too little sleep means the body does not have enough time to renew itself.

Just like stress, insufficient sleep also impacts all 11 body systems and creates a cascade of issues. These are some of the negative physiological issues that result from insufficient sleep:

- **Circulatory system:** When people don't sleep, they're more prone to cardiovascular disease and hypertension and have an increased risk of stroke and heart attack.

- **Endocrine system:** Lack of sleep contributes to problems with the body responding properly to the hormone insulin. Insulin regulates blood sugar levels. Over time, this increases the risk of developing type 2 diabetes.

---

107 "Five Fascinating Historical Sleep Facts," Dormeo, accessed March 13, 2024, https://www.dormeo.co.uk/blog/sleep-science/five-fascinating-historical-sleep-facts.

- **Gastrointestinal system:** When we don't sleep, it disrupts our hormones that regulate our appetite. This leads to hunger and weight gain.

- **Immune system:** Insomnia suppresses the body's immune system's production of virus-killing cells. When we don't sleep enough, our risk of getting ill dramatically increases.

- **Integumentary system:** Lack of sleep dampens the healing action of collagen, the fibrous protein found in the body's connective tissues. This means you age prematurely.

- **Muscular system:** When we don't sleep well, it impedes the muscular system's ability to replace, repair, and rebuild itself.

- **Nervous system:** Not sleeping enough compromises the brain's executive functions. This impairs cognitive skills such as concentration, memory, and the regulation of emotions. If this goes on for an extended period of time, it will lead to mood swings, anxiety, and depression.

- **Renal/urinary system:** Lack of sleep interrupts the pattern of the body's rhythm of urination and enhances levels of nighttime urinary output.

- **Reproductive system:** If we don't sleep well, it can even dampen sex drive and lower reproductive hormone levels in both men and women. This causes fertility issues.

- **Respiratory system:** Trouble snoozing boosts the incidence of respiratory illness and intensifies the symptoms of chronic lung disease.

- **Skeletal system:** Lack of shut-eye even attacks our bones. It decreases bone density and bone marrow composition.[108]

---

108 Frates et al., *Lifestyle Medicine Handbook.*

That's a dump truck full of negative health consequences waiting to zap us if we don't catch enough zzz's. It's not surprising that the one-third of adults complaining about tossing and turning during the night turn to health-care providers to help them.[109]

There's a lot of emerging research that cognitive behavioral therapy is greatly beneficial in tackling insomnia.[110] That includes mindfulness and relaxation exercises, as we explored in chapter 7, and working with our natural sleeping rhythms.[111]

For me, though, cognitive behavioral therapy wasn't a grand slam to restoring my sleeping pattern. Weary, yet still clinging to hope that sleep was possible for me, I dove into my ever-trusty YouTube. I found podcasts on sleep and discovered the world of "sleep hygiene." For those of us who aren't sleep scientists, that means "healthy habits for sleep preparation." This includes watching out for and stopping sneaky sleep thieves.

Sleep Thieves

- Anxiety
- Depression
- Sedentary lifestyle
- Medications
- Illness and pain
- Perimenopause/menopause

- Electronic devices
- Caffeine
- Alcohol
- Nicotine
- Heavy meals
- Obesity

---

109 Cristina Mutchler, "Insomnia Facts and Statistics: What You Need to Know," Verywell Health, September 15, 2022, https://www.verywellhealth.com/insomnia-facts-and-statistics-5498718.

110 "Insomnia Treatment: Cognitive Behavioral Therapy instead of Sleeping Pills," Mayo Clinic, April 5, 2023, https://www.mayoclinic.org/diseases-conditions/insomnia/in-depth/insomnia-treatment/art-20046677.

111 Rachel Zoffness, *The Pain Management Workbook: Powerful CBT and Mindfulness Skills to Take Control of Pain and Reclaim Your Life* (Oakland, CA: New Harbinger Publications, 2020).

- Sleep apnea
- Jet lag
- Noisy sleeping conditions

If any of these culprits are present in your life like they were in mine, you may be experiencing:

- Fatigue

- Irritability

- Anxiety

- Depression

- Poor concentration or memory

Well, I had serious no-nos that I was going to have to stop—like using my tablet in bed when I was awake at 2 a.m. Oops. But even though I stopped doing the sleep-robbing activities, my sleep only improved slightly. Like a child looking for the stash of hidden Halloween treats, I kept exploring the research for more answers.

Finally, one glorious fall morning, I found the treasure trove. I learned the body has to wind down from alert to full-on sleep. It's a whole orchestra of systems in action that need to shift gears. Scientists found that stopping stimulating the brain a few hours before you hit the hay aids the body in winding down into sleep.[112]

The general advice for getting good sleep includes:

- **Keep a Regular Schedule:** That means going to bed and waking up the same time every day, even on weekends and holidays.

- **Cultivate a Comfortable Environment:** Make sure your bedroom

---

112 "Insomnia Treatment."

is quiet, dark, and a comfortable temperature. If necessary, use blackout curtains and white noise machines. Also, make sure you are sleeping on a mattress and pillows that work for your anatomy.

- **Limit Screen Time:** Avoid screens at least an hour before bed, as the blue light emitted can interfere with production of melatonin, the hormone that signals that it's time to sleep.

- **Use Relaxation Techniques:** Do activities and routines that are relaxing and help you wind down before bed.

- **Get Physical Exercise:** Exercise promotes better sleep if done during the day and not too close to bedtime.

- **Watch Caffeine:** Caffeine stays in the system for a long time, so stop drinking it at least four to six hours before bedtime.

As I looked at the list, I came up with guidelines that I needed to apply. For me, that meant that I stopped drinking caffeine in the afternoons after 3 p.m. and didn't comment on social media in the evenings. It also meant that, when the sun faded, it was time to tuck away my technology, including the tablet and phone, for the night. The blue light that comes from them stimulates the brain to be awake.

I also made a ritual of soaking in a lavender-scented Epsom salt bath with classical music playing in the background in the early evening. In the tub, I'd enjoy savoring the flavor of decaffeinated teas while I leafed through magazines I had neglected due to my binge usage of my iPad.

For actual sleeping time, I made my bedroom a sleep sanctuary, where sleep dreams ran wild. I learned the power of dark drapes (often called blackout curtains). The drapes block out streetlights for the city folks and limit the glare of the moonlight so the darkness signals the brain that it's time to rest. Amazingly, they also help with regulating room temperatures through the change of the seasons. Plus, the added privacy helps people feel more relaxed. Not only did I hang beautiful sage curtains to serve this purpose, but I also removed my clock to keep things nice and cave-like.

All of these helped as a starting point, and I did manage to clock a few more hours, but to truly achieve the kind of sleep I wanted, I had to uplevel even more and research deeper findings.

Case Study: Chaplain Bonnie Learns to Sleep Through the Night (Yep, It's Me Again ☺)

I had a wealth of scientific information on how to fix my sleep, but I needed to come up with a game plan to shift my brain into the world of sleep.

Here's my personalized system I created for myself in addition to the advice I shared above.

1. Walk in the Fresh Air Every Day

The exhilaration of being in the fresh air and the release of endorphins reduces stress and calms the mind. The increased oxygen exchange strengthens the immune system. Engaging in moderate outdoor exercise increases the body's need for rest. It's also a great time to soak in natural sunlight (a source of vitamin D). The vitamin D helps regulate the body's circadian rhythms, which act as the body's internal clock. It synchronizes the sleep-wake cycle roughly every 24 hours.

2. Stop Eating after 6 p.m.

When we eat, the body needs to digest the food. This increases its metabolic activity and body temperature. High-calorie meals can impair the quality of rest. Eating too close to bedtime has been shown to increase the number of awakenings at night and reduce the amount of deep sleep.[113] Restricting food at night aids in weight management and reduces the risk of disorders such as sleep apnea.

3. Reduce Beverages in the Evening

To cut back on disturbances, reduce your liquids two to three hours before bedtime. This should decrease how often you need to do the middle-of-the-night run to the restroom. In order to remain healthy while implementing this strategy, make sure to focus on drinking enough water during the earlier part of the day to prevent dehydration. To determine the best cutoff time, experiment and track what works best for your body.

4. Refrain from Napping During the Day

Okay, did I attack your favorite activity? Don't worry. Short naps have been found to have a lot of benefits. What you want to watch out for is long naps or snoozing too close to bedtime. Unfortunately, these two behaviors disrupt the sleep-wake cycle and make a good night's sleep hard to snatch.

5. Remember That the Bedroom Is for Sleep and Sex Only

Our brains form connections between different environments and the activities we perform there.[114] If we work in a space, our minds will more likely associate that space with our professional responsibilities, potentially leading to increased stress when we spend time there.

---

113 Frates et al., *Lifestyle Medicine Handbook.*
114 Frates et al., *Lifestyle Medicine Handbook.*

I made it a rule for myself to maintain a sleep- and sex-friendly environment in my bedroom. No work, and I keep it clean and clutter-free to promote tranquil sleep and passionate sex.

6. Turn Off the Tablet an Hour before Bedtime and Leave the Phone in the Other Room

Tablets and mobile phones send out a blue light that fools the brain into thinking it's daylight, regardless of the time. The blue light messes with our melatonin production. Also, our dang phones and electronic devices are designed to keep us engaged. This is the opposite of what we need to be doing to relax before hitting the sack. Remember, the goal is not to swipe right but to transition into unwinding.

Part of that unwinding is to say no to work, emails, and news. All of that can wait. As an added bonus of getting away from our devices, we aren't disturbed by the notifications and sounds those devices like to make that can jolt us from sleep.

Advanced tip: Most devices have built-in features to dim that annoying blue light. You can schedule regular evening downtime for blue light emissions that will help protect your sleep if you just can't stay off technology.

If you have to use a screen before bedtime, you can minimize the blue light messing with your melatonin by wearing special blue-light-blocking glasses. There are many different types of blue-light-blocking glasses. You can order prescription glasses with specific blue-light-blocking coatings or tints.

When you search for blue-light-blocking glasses, it's easy to get overwhelmed. There are many different choices in color tint. According to some experts, the tint color does matter.

The company BlockBlueLight claims that:

- **Clear glasses** are for the daytime with computer and device use.

- **Yellow glasses** are also for daytime use if you are prone to headaches and migraines. The yellow is also supposed to guard against eye damage.

- **Amber glasses** are for the evening to reduce stress and keep the circadian rhythm working for you.

- **Red glasses** are the bomb, protecting you 100% from the nasty dangers of blue light emissions and giving you the best sleep. [115]

Another option is over-the-counter blue-light-blocking glasses. These glasses are designed in a style that can be worn alone if you don't need glasses, but they can also fit over prescription glasses.

7. Establish Consistent Times to Go to Bed and Wake Up

A consistent sleep schedule is magic to our body. By having a regular schedule, the body can count on our body's circadian rhythm and heart rate, blood pressure, and other cardiovascular functions to stay smooth and steady. This gives our internal clock a chance to establish a restorative sleeping pattern.

8. Stop All Work After 6 p.m. and Shift into Relaxation Activities

Having a cutoff time to stop focusing on work assists in shifting our minds to relaxing activities. For me, because my bedtime is 10 p.m. to accommodate my *exceedingly* early morning meetings, I picked 6 p.m. for my cutoff time.

---

115 "Blue Light Lens Colour Guide," BlockBlueLight, accessed October 18, 2023, https://www.blockbluelight.co.uk/pages/blue-light-lens-colour-guide.

My husband and I are empty nesters, so I don't have any evening parenting duties. I get to spend my evenings playing with my birds, making jewelry, or creating one-of-a-kind blouses and skirts.

9. Stop Scrolling and Responding on Social Media by 5 p.m., Even on the Weekends

My social media is related to work and my other passions. So, okay, I admit it. There are times I can become highly involved in responding to people struggling with chronic pain. I save this for earlier in the day, when I have more energy and it doesn't interfere with a good night's sleep.

10. Engage in Activities That Relax You Instead of Watching TV

Some people wouldn't even consider TV before bed; they find it more soothing to select a book with an interesting topic, listen to gentle music, or do light stretching to relax, rather than hearing disturbing news. Other people enjoy getting late-night news or watching shows before bed. Whichever group you fall into, though, it's important to remember that TV is a bad choice before bed because of the blue light that messes with our internal clock. Unfortunately, binge-watching shows wakes the body up rather than calming it.

11. Perform Mindfulness Exercises Before Bedtime

Practicing deep breathing and listening to relaxation videos that stimulate the relaxation responses are great to do right before bed. Our body collects tension throughout the day. These exercises steer the mind away from racing thoughts and lull it into a calm state that slows the heart, breathing, and thoughts.

12. Refrain from Talking on the Phone in the Evenings

Although I enjoy chatting with family and friends, it stimulates my mind and requires mental and emotional engagement that I've found is difficult to wind down from. And let's face it, though I'm always interested to hear people share the twists and turns of their lives, I'm at my best responding to their challenges when I'm refreshed after a good night's sleep.

If you work during the day so evening is the only time to talk with your family, focus on staying in a calm state while you connect with your loved ones. This will enable you to shift to sleep mode at the end of your evening.

By putting away my phone, I stay away from the blue light and disconnect from outside stimulus so I can just be. I've found this to be extremely beneficial for getting a good night's sleep, which contributes to my overall health.

13. Keep a Sleep Journal and Wear a Fitness Tracker

Each night before I go to sleep, I jot down notes in my sleep journal about my evening activities, including how many beverages I drank and what they were, what time I started preparing for bed, and what I did to down-regulate my body.

In the morning, I immediately check my Fitbit (a fitness tracker). This device tracks hours slept and how much of that sleep was deep sleep. This gives me a good idea of the quality of sleep I'm getting. I also review the notes in my journal to see the impact of my sleep habits from the night before.

As you can see, my personal 13-step sleep-friendly program wasn't a quick fix, but each step helped improve my sleeping patterns. In fact, miracle of miracles, not only do I now enjoy sweet slumber, but it's getting easier and easier to ease myself into dreamland. When I wake up in the middle of the night, I'm able to go back to sleep by reaching for an electrically heated eye mask and practicing deep breathing and relaxation exercises. I now clock between six and seven hours of sleep every night. Many aches have disappeared, my mood has improved, and my body has made huge leaps on its healing journey.

What I love about these solutions is how affordable making these changes can be. For less than the price of visiting a sleep clinic, I purchased room-darkening curtains, a budget fitness tracker, and an electric eye mask.

To plan your sleep improvement system, it's important to remember:

- Don't keep a tablet or phone in your bedroom.

- Don't engage in vigorous exercise like cardio workouts or high-intensity interval training two hours before bedtime. If your schedule requires you to exercise at night, remember that your body needs time to down-regulate. Adjusting your bedtime to a later hour can help you achieve a good night's sleep.

- Don't drink caffeinated beverages late in the afternoon. This includes organic caffeinated drinks.

- Don't eat a full meal late in the evening because digesting food close to bedtime can disrupt your sleep.

- Don't nap longer than 20 minutes so your body will sleep better at bedtime.

- Avoid stimulating conversation prior to bedtime.

- Don't watch emotionally stimulating shows close to bedtime.

- Don't sleep in to make up for lost sleep. It's important to maintain a consistent wake and sleep schedule to help your internal clock stay in a healing rhythm.

In this chapter, we learned how sleep impacts our total health and can aggravate pain conditions. There are many behavioral changes you can undertake to achieve a better sleep pattern.

In the next chapter, you'll learn how social connections are important for our physical and emotional well-being and how, despite having chronic pain, you can still stay socially connected.

REMEMBER:

- Sleep impacts all 11 biological systems.

- Adequate sleep is essential to minimize pain and to help the body heal.

- It's important to remember to shift the body into sleep mode each night.

- You can improve your sleep by conscientiously practicing positive sleep hygiene behaviors.

CHAPTER 14

The Healing Power of Social Connections

♥

"Only through our connectedness to others can we really know and enhance the self."
—HARRIET GOLDHOR LERNER, CLINICAL PSYCHOLOGIST

O n March 20, 2020, I glanced out my front window in the middle of a brisk day and saw bundled-up parents dashing to the elementary school next door. The parents were wearing frowns as they hurried along.

Something was wrong.

I snatched my jacket on my way out of my house and asked a passing mom, "What's happening?"

"An order just went out to immediately close down all the schools," the young mom yelled out to me, still continuing toward the school. She said over her shoulder, "It's the COVID pandemic."

When I had studied the 1918 flu pandemic in my epidemiology (study of the distribution and causes of diseases and conditions) class, I'd read about pandemics. In class we had seen black-and-white photos of "closed" signs on schools, businesses, and places of worship under headlines with grim death statistics.

After hearing that COVID was the reason for the early school closure, I hurried back inside the house and immediately turned on the local news for an update. Our region needed to hunker down to stay safe until scientists figured out how to tame the virus. This meant that all bookstores, coffee shops, gyms, libraries, and even some grocery stores were closing due to concern for the welfare of their employees.

Snapping off the television, I headed to Len's office, where he was busy working.

"It happened." That earned a cursory glance from him while he continued debugging a complex computer program.

"Businesses and schools are closing due to the pandemic." I dropped this news bomb for him to absorb. "A stay-at-home order has been issued."

As he took in the news, I considered the impact it was going to have on the memorial service that I was scheduled to officiate that upcoming weekend. It would have to be canceled, and I didn't look forward to making that call to the bereaved family.

"I've got to get busy canceling all my in-person appointments and memorials until further notice," I moaned.

Len's fingers continued dancing on the keyboard. He stared at me with a blank face. "How're *you* going to handle being home all the time?"

"I'm going to be fine. I'm used to being at home. Years of experience. I'll use my phone to do my chaplaincy check-ins, and I'll only schedule online video memorials until it's safe to gather in groups."

He gave an ever-so-slight shake of his head. "We both know you'll go crazy not being around people."

"I did it for three decades." I shrugged. "This will not be a problem."

He raised his eyebrows at my declaration.

"Time to feed the parrots," I said, committed to showing him I was right.

For the first few weeks of March, being housebound was okay—meaning, I distracted myself by instituting a morning text check-in with people in my life. After that, I got busy developing materials for my future in-person pain management workshops. In the background, I'd listen to the latest COVID news reporting on the growing number of communities hit hard by the disease.

We were experiencing a shortage of pasta, rice, canned goods, and produce due to the pandemic disrupting the global supply chain. When it became clear that things weren't going to return to normal any time soon, I turned to YouTube to watch World War II food rationing cooking shows, searching for ideas for creating yummy meals based on what I had in my pantry.

As a chaplain, I was very aware of the increasing stress that was rising with parents juggling work and having their children at home. The kids had become extremely restless, especially preschoolers, who didn't have the structure of having their teachers online that their older brothers and sisters did. My friend who was the director of a preschool shared her concern about her stuck-at-home students and asked if I could create YouTube puppet and parrot shows to bring some joy into her students' lives. I jumped at the opportunity.

Not only did I get to play with the puppets I'd been collecting since my days as a police chaplain, but this also gave me a chance to use my creativity to make the children laugh and learn about health and stress all at the same time. Bingo!

My days were filled with writing children's scripts and recruiting my most cooperative parrots into my primitive sound studio. When I'd star in the show, I'd take off my most sparkly necklaces to guard against any parrot theft attempts. I also made sure to keep the wires to my newly purchased lapel microphone hidden from their curious beaks.

Family members reported that during the show, their kids would giggle, clap, and yell at the screen for the puppets and parrots to do and say things. A mom and her kids sent me a video thank-you and expressed their appreciation that I had created the show. That inspired me to post an advertisement for the show in my front yard.

My neighbors started to share the videos with their young grandkids, nieces, and nephews across the country. A request arrived asking me to do a show about food allergies for their four-year-old, who had been recently diagnosed with a peanut allergy. After I created the video, I sent them a special note telling the family that the next time they visited our town, they had a standing invitation to meet my parrots and puppets.

I was flying high from the boost of dopamine I got from the impact of my creative efforts. My mornings were packed with a fury of activity as I researched early childhood stress management tips to craft into scripts. By afternoon each day, I was looking for a break, and social media beckoned me to spend hours mindlessly scrolling through funny parrot and one-of-a-kind jewelry postings on Instagram and Facebook. I fought the impulse to continue into the night, knowing it would hurt my sleep.

Even though I was having a good time with these activities, the gray walls of my house closed in on me as my husband was working remotely, only peeking his head out for food. I found myself having conversations with my parrots, who mostly said, "Bye-bye."

Message received.

My flock's snubbing me drove me to beg Len to accompany me on my daily after-lunch hike around our neighborhood. He's a quiet, thoughtful type of guy who lives in his head, but on our first climb up the hill, he enthusiastically described a new computer program he was creating.

I was able to follow his incredibly detailed description as I huffed and puffed, trying to keep up with his long strides. Catching my breath, I gasped out a name for his new program. From then on, to keep me happy, he squeezed in a daily afternoon pandemic outing. First we'd discuss his computer programming, and then we would shift to my newest script for the children who were suffering from missing their schoolmates. This didn't seem to hold his interest, outside of asking about the ins and outs of uploading my videos on YouTube.

A few days after instituting our daily ritual, I was running out of descriptions of the technical side of YouTube, so I decided I needed to play Scheherazade, the clever Middle Eastern storyteller from the book *One Thousand and One Nights*. My goal was to weave captivating stories based on the health impact of positive social connections with cliffhangers to capture my husband's attention and keep him willing to walk.

To do this, I investigated the health impact of positive social connections. I dove into creating colorful personalities for my daily stories using science-based information. I told him the data of the research and left out what it meant.

Remarkably, he actually slowed his pace as he got busy making connections and working toward solutions. The man couldn't resist a good puzzle. He connected the dots that having friends in one's life drastically improved one's physical and mental health. Soon after our walks began, he reconnected with his old friends. (Yes, he became more fun to live with, so for sure there was a hidden agenda woven into my stories.)

The American Psychological Association (APA) defines loneliness as "The emotional distress we feel when our inherent needs for intimacy and companionship are not met." Loneliness is a risk factor for developing depression, and it takes a toll on the body.[116]

Many people with chronic pain have to frequently cancel social engagements, which may cause their social lives to fade. It's easy to see in this situation how loneliness can grow to the point where a person's only social interactions include trips to the pharmacy or to medical appointments, especially if they are no longer able to work.

A study by Cigna noted that loneliness was on the rise before the pandemic hit, with 61% of Americans reporting being lonely in 2019. This was up from 54% of people who reported being lonely in 2018.[117]

Many articles suggested that the jump was in part due to increased mobility. Moving led people to lose their established social networks. Others experienced a decrease in face-to-face social interactions due to reliance on emails and texting. Still others were hit by economic troubles that caused them to isolate. On a social level, you might have noticed that more people are now comfortable discussing personal issues than people have been in the past. This has caused people to be more aware of their feelings of loneliness and has made them more willing to admit to having that struggle.

---

116 Carmen Chai, "All About Loneliness: What Causes it, How to Cope With It, and When to Get Help," Everyday Health, July 29, 2022, https://www.everydayhealth.com/loneliness/.
117 Lindsay Modglin, "What Is Loneliness? Causes, Effects and Prevention," Forbes Health, February 20, 2023, https://www.forbes.com/health/mind/what-is-loneliness/.

We're wired in our DNA for connection, and it's essential for overall well-being. Even if you don't consider yourself a "people person," when you interact with others, either in person, by phone, or through Zoom, your brain releases feel-good neurotransmitters, producing feelings of happiness, connectedness, and pleasure.

The research lit a passion in me to deepen my connections and to serve those who I knew were suffering in a bigger way. I started sharing a daily count "sheltering in place" timeline along with an uplifting essay about emotional and physical health on both Instagram and Facebook.

"This is Chaplain Bonnie signing off on this ___ day of sheltering in place" was the opening line for my writing, which I continued to do for 14 straight months. The first night that I hit the key that shared my posts simultaneously to Instagram and Facebook, I held my breath, wondering if people would respond to my count timeline and story.

My eyes lit up when, within minutes, people from all over the world left comments about how wonderful it was to read uplifting words in the middle of the terror of COVID. Warm waves of relief went through me. From that day on, I received private messages from people telling me how much they looked forward to reading my posts.

Not only did this countdown connect others, but it also connected me to the bigger world. It gave me and my readers the sense of community and the rush of happy chemicals that our brains needed to make the shelter in place more of a comfortable experience.

All the activities I engaged in during the pandemic made a huge differ-ence in my life and made me a believer in the importance of having ties to others. Maybe you're feeling that it might be hard for you to build and maintain connections when you're in so much pain that every fiber in your body is shouting at you, or maybe you don't even think that you require social connections, but guess what? Research says you would feel better with friendly contacts, and your health would benefit.[118]

Maybe you think that you are okay because you are in a relationship with a partner. But research has proven over and over again that interacting with a variety of people contributes to new experiences and helps maintain a sense of individuality and independence.[119] Plus, wouldn't it be nice to indulge in that one thing your partner doesn't like with other people who share your passion?

When it comes to building connection with others, it's important to consider that we each have different ways to meet these needs. One person might feel like she's a social butterfly after lunching with a friend once a month. Another person may enjoy weekly movie dates and group chair yoga class at least three times a week, followed by lunch dates. Still others consider that watching the game with neighbors just about does it.

Although each of us has social needs, the level of those needs varies. Also, it's important to consider that we have different energy levels depending on where we are in our healing journey.

I'm known as an entertaining storyteller who can comfortably chat for hours, but I'm overwhelmed by planning lunch dates. The important thing is to select the social interactions that you enjoy doing.

If your chronic pain makes going out challenging, there are plenty of activities you can do from the comfort of your home. Below are just a few ideas to consider. Choose the ones that ignite your interests.

- Reach out to someone you genuinely like by phone, Zoom or other

118 "Friendships: Enrich Your Life and Improve Your Health," Mayo Clinic, January 12, 2022, https://www.mayoclinic.org/healthy-lifestyle/adult-health/in-depth/friendships/art-20044860.
119 April Eldemire, "Why Friendships Are Vital to the Health of Your Relationship," Psychology Today, May 30, 2019, https://www.psychologytoday.com/us/blog/couples-thrive/201905/why-friendships-are-vital-the-health-your-relationship.

video chat, in person, or via texting and emailing.

- Perform random acts of kindness, such as anonymously sending a gift card or shipping a book to a family member or friend. This allows for a no-strings-attached interaction as you wade into the process of creating social connections.

- Volunteer for an hour or two at an animal shelter, food bank, house of worship, childcare center, hospital, library, or local museum. If you're experiencing a flare-up, you can still volunteer from bed. On social media platforms, you can share informative content and engage in discussions about issues or organizations you support. Other opportunities include online mentoring, tutoring, or providing emotional support through text or email.

- Smile at people on Zoom.

- Give hearts to social media posts.

- Check in on a senior or a young parent.

- Smile and nod to people when you take walks. Use a compliment about their dog, child, or sporty outfit to open the door to an interesting conversation.

- Join a walking group or low-impact exercise program.

- Participate in your community's recreation and leisure activities, such as outdoor concerts and community festivals.

- Greet cashiers at stores you frequent or say hi to the person who drops off your food orders or groceries. Everyone likes to be acknowledged and share their thoughts about the weather.

- Sign up for Zoom and Meetup hobby classes like cooking, gardening, and expressive arts. It's a great way to meet new people.

- Start or join a book club, either online or in person.

- Go to a coffee shop and read books and take notes on important passages. (As I mentioned in chapter 6, I did this and regulars thought I was an author and would chat with me.)

- Connect online through support groups.

- Attend services at your place of worship and participate in their sponsored social activities.

- Sign up for a plot at your town's community garden.

- Walk your neighbor's dog (this changed my life) or take a stroll with a grandchild, child, spouse, friend, or even by yourself.

- Attend a relevant 12-step group, either in person or online.

Case Study: Ankylosing Spondylitis

On an early August morning, I pulled up my bathing suit and adjusted the straps. I glanced at the clock to see if I was on schedule and suddenly remembered to grab my thin nylon zip-up swim jacket. Due to my history of CRPS, my body is hypersensitive to drafts when I'm in the water. Wearing the jacket over my swimsuit keeps my shoulder muscles from aching from drafts most people don't notice.

That morning, I was embarking on my first ever "Water Walking with the Chaplain" at our city's natatorium (the fancy Latin word for an indoor swimming pool). Water walking is a wonderful exercise for chronic pain conditions. Strolling through the water and swinging your arms against the resistance is a great way to exercise the body without aggravating your joints. It can be performed in a leisurely way by beginners or aerobically for those who can tolerate a more challenging workout.

The early morning sky had an orange tint due to the raging forest fires in

Northern California. Our air quality was still in the healthy range in those early days of our fire season. I took in the beauty of the sky as I drove to meet Dorothy. After weeks of phone-based meetings, I was finally going to meet this 65-year-old retired elementary school teacher who suffered from ankylosing spondylitis and had a keen interest in reading literacy. She infused her love of literature, especially Jane Austen, Shakespeare, and other classic literature, into every conversation. No matter what we discussed, she always amazed me when she referred to an author's work that covered our topic.

Ankylosing Spondylitis

Ankylosing spondylitis (AS) is a type of arthritis that favors men two to three times more than women. No matter who it decides to invade, the symptoms are the same—inflammation in the joints and ligaments of the spine. This inflammation creates stiffness and, in severe cases, the joints fuse. The condition ranges from mild infrequent episodes of back pain and stiffness to a severe condition that contributes to a chronic pain situation.[120] In the most severe cases, the hips, ribs, shoulders, knees, ankles, and feet can be affected by the disease.

Anyone can develop AS. The cause is unknown and there is no known cure.

Symptoms

- Pain, stiffness, and inflammation in joints

- Difficulty inhaling deeply if ribs are affected

- Vision changes due to inflammation in the eye

- Fatigue

- Loss of appetite and weight loss

---

120 "Ankylosing Spondylitis," National Institute of Arthritis and Musculoskeletal and Skin Diseases, accessed March 13, 2024, https://www.niams.nih.gov/health-topics/ankylosing-spondylitis.

- Skin rashes

- Stomach pain and loose bowel movements[121]

Risk Factors

- **Genetics:** Family history of this disease increases the risk.

- **Age:** Most people are diagnosed before age 45. AS may affect adolescents and children.

- **Other conditions:** People with Crohn's disease, ulcerative colitis, or psoriasis are more prone to this type of arthritis.[122]

Diagnosis

- Medical and family history

- Physical exam

- Imaging studies

- Lab tests

Treatments

- Medications, including NSAIDs, Enbrel, and Humira to relieve inflammation and accompanying stiffness and reduce complications like spinal deformity[123]

- Physical therapy to maintain range of motion and strengthen abdominal muscles

- Self-management activities

121 "Ankylosing Spondylitis."
122 "Ankylosing Spondylitis."
123 Ali Gies, "Ankylosing Spondylitis Progression: What to Expect," MySpondylitisTeam, last updated December 27, 2022, https://www.myspondylitisteam.com/resources/the-progression-of-ankylosing-spondylitis.

- Stay active by walking to maintain flexibility and improve posture

- Don't smoke

- Maintain healthy weight

- Manage stress

- Get adequate sleep

- Stay socially connected

Dorothy had reached out to me through a neighborhood app after seeing a post about my upcoming community health event about how to improve your quality of life. Her chief concerns were her deteriorating health and feeling down from stressful life events. Hearing that I worked one-on-one with clients, she had asked if she could schedule a meeting with me.

In the previous two years, she had retired from a much-loved elementary school teaching career, welcomed her first grandchild, and faced the tragic passing of her husband. They had just celebrated their fortieth anniversary when he was taken by lung cancer.

Crushed by his passing and unable to keep up with the demands of managing the family's two-story home, Dorothy had moved to a neighboring town and settled into a sleek single-story two-bedroom condo closer to shopping and transportation.

Dorothy told me that she preferred to talk on the phone rather than meet through Zoom. She explained she didn't feel comfortable on camera due to her place still being full of boxes that she hadn't been able to unpack due to her aching body.

She was experiencing intermittent pain and stiffness in her lower back and found herself tossing and turning throughout the nights. Every morning, she woke feeling like a low battery in desperate need of a recharge. Adding to that, a sadness had hovered over her since she had left her old neighborhood where she had lived with her husband, raised her children, and led a lively book club for over 20 years.

"I can only imagine how your mind must be reeling from all the changes in your life," I said after she finished her update.

She gave a big sigh.

"I love my bright new condo, but my life has changed so much." She added, "I guess it's time to take a look at a book my husband read a long time ago about coping with change. It's called *Who Moved My Cheese?*"

Her book reference was perfect since it explored mindsets people can have when faced with change and presented coping skills. The fact that she was referring to a book about change suggested she'd be open to doing things differently.

"Did you know that stress, loneliness, and lack of sleep create problems not only for chronic pain patients, but for all people experiencing these issues?" I asked, diving right in.

"I thought it was the inflammation of AS raising its ugly head stopping me from making my new place a home. It hurts too much to mount my family photos or put out my collection of Lalique glass vases and perfume bottles."

"I'm sure that's part of it, but lack of sleep makes your muscles and bones ache even more. Would you like to learn the facts about how to wake up feeling refreshed?"

She laughed. "To paraphrase Danielle Steel, 'I'll celebrate the joy of learning as long as I live.'"

Capitalizing on her positive attitude, we dove into exploring her sleep habits. She bought an Apple watch on eBay to monitor the quality of her sleep. It quickly became evident that playing solitaire on her iPad in bed every night was disrupting her sleep pattern. The tablet had been an anniversary gift from her late husband. She found the act of strategically building piles of cards in ascending order strangely addicting and calming, and it helped her feel close to him.

When she learned that the blue light generated by the screen on her device activated her nervous system and reduced melatonin, she knew she had to give it up. Still wanting to feel close to her husband, though, she chose to use her iPad during the day to stream music, and instead of flipping cards electronically, she invested in a deck of cards and played solitaire on a dinner tray in her bed. Within a few nights of doing that, she found she could only play a few hands before her eyes drooped shut.

During our subsequent phone chats, she told me that she was sleeping better and feeling better. Now that she had more strength, we discussed the stresses of widowhood. Fortunately, she and her husband had paid attention to estate planning, so she didn't have the headache of dealing with probate, but she had a huge amount of stress from managing her finances for the first time.

She was in the middle of obsessively sharing her worries when I gently interrupted her, saying, "When you worry and say you can't handle things, it churns up negative chemicals that increase your pain."

Silence came from her end of the phone.

I used that as an opportunity to give her a short overview of how stress impacts the body by not only causing emotional upset but also increasing tension in muscle groups, disrupting the digestive system, and dampening down the body's immune system's ability to fight off illnesses.

"One way I like to counter stress is by writing down my stressors. Once they're all listed out, I brainstorm ideas to deal with them," I said. "Looking for solutions stimulates neurotransmitters that make me feel better."

"I can do that," she said.

A few weeks later, she shared that she'd created a special graphic for her stressors and possible solutions. She had used construction paper and selected different colors to represent each stressor to create a pie chart. The most pressing stressors were cut into the largest wedges. One was labeled "finances," the next one "health," and then "grief." After pasting all the wedges on a poster board, she titled it, "Stressors to Manage."

She displayed her stress board on her living room wall alongside a list of techniques to manage them. Her goal was to whittle down each wedge. Every day she'd tackle her finances, health, and her lingering grief by experimenting with strategies to find out which ones worked the best.

Over the next few weeks, her pie wedges changed in both nature and number as her focus shifted and the problems became more manageable. The day finally arrived when things worked well enough for her that she changed the labels on the wedges to "friends," "fun exercises," and "books I want to read." Her goal was now to ensure that she paid attention to these areas that she now knew made her happy.

All of this made her more confident about making day-to-day decisions. Even though she had started doing some social activities, she held back because she was missing her old friends. She had mentioned several times that she felt too old to make new friends. So, when she mentioned that her physical therapist had suggested water walking to improve her range of motion and overall strength, I saw it as an opportunity to support her not only with her physical health but also with her deep loneliness.

"I love water walking," I said quickly. "You don't get your hair wet, and you get to chat with people. What can be better than that?"

"Well, I don't know. I would feel kind of funny."

"Would it make it better if I went with you?"

"Yes!"

The next day, I found myself at the pool scanning the deck for Dorothy, who said she'd be wearing a black swimsuit decorated with bird-of-paradise flowers. I waved at her, and she laughed when she saw that my swim jacket had a coral Hawaiian hibiscus splashed across the front. Not only did we discover that the two of us had Hawaiian-themed beachwear in common, but both of us are on the short side with bobbed graying hair and love to talk a mile a minute.

After we hugged, she said, "It looks like we're on a tropical vacation."

I scoured the pool area. "Except there's no banyan trees, and our sky outside is being lit up by the raging forest fires up north."

The condensation droplets on the floor-to-ceiling windows that surrounded the pool made it appear as if we were peering through a kaleidoscope. The sun's rays filtered through the smoke and filled the horizon with swatches of orange and pink. The powdered ash from the fire that coated the cars in the northern Bay Area hadn't yet reached our valley.

We approached the shallow indoor walking pool, breathing in chlorine. Cautiously, we stepped down onto the pool's wide cement steps into surprisingly comfortable water. After we luxuriated in it for a few moments, we walked the length of the pool to loosen up our muscles. I suggested that we swing our arms through the water to increase our heart rate.

Just as I suspected would happen, other women walkers joined in, talking with us. We soon learned that everyone in our pool had either a bad back or arthritis. One of the ladies told Dorothy that she should consider joining the natatorium's group water aerobics class that met four times a week. She added that the exercises were gentle and many participants had bad backs or osteoarthritis.

On the way out of the pool, Dorothy stopped at the front desk to grab information about the water aerobics class. One of our co–water walkers mentioned that many of the water aerobics class members went for coffee after every class, and we were more than welcome to join them.

Dorothy quickly became a regular at the natatorium, where she enjoyed the comfort of the water and new friends. She was even recruited to read for the children's reading hour at the local library.

Our last check-in happened in October at the end of our fire season. Though it would be weeks before we saw our first rain, the region's air quality had improved. As we sat chatting in the coffee shop, we weren't surprised that we both personally knew people who had experienced the trauma of losing their homes in the fires.

Dorothy shook her head. "It seemed like every week a new video showed frantic people driving through walls of flames."

Despite that sad news, we celebrated that Dorothy's overall discomfort with AS had decreased due in part to her gentle exercises and her newfound ability to sleep at least six hours every night.

Personally, I suspected that her new friends and social life played an even bigger role in minimizing her discomfort. The importance of social connections is one of my most favorite topics to discuss because of the dramatic impact that occurs when it is effectively nurtured. The strategies shared in this chapter have worked for many people to instill joy in their lives. I hope you'll be implementing some of them to warm your heart today. We can all use more friends.

In the following chapter, you'll explore the value of developing a positive collaborative relationship with your physicians and therapists. You'll also learn how to transform yourself from being seen just as a medical diagnostic number by learning how to develop a checklist that will improve your communication with your health-care providers, whether during an office visit or an online appointment. And finally, you'll learn how to manage viewing your online records and lab work results.

REMEMBER:

- Social connections are necessary for our physical and mental well-being.

- We are biologically programmed to be social.

- Social connections help stimulate our feel-good chemicals.

- In spite of living with chronic pain, there are many avenues to stay connected with others.

- Individuals have different levels of need for social connections due to their personalities and energy levels.

CHAPTER 15

Ramp Up Your Health Team to Keep You Healing

♥

"An average doctor saves a body; a good doctor saves a being."

—ABHIJIT NASKAR, NEUROSCIENTIST

In the 1960s, I grew up watching the medical drama *Dr. Kildare*. The show followed the extremely good-looking Richard Chamberlain as his character wrestled with the moral issues medicine brings up. He bravely fought for the best health of his patients.

There was also *Marcus Welby, M.D.* Granted, Robert Young was not as good-looking as dreamy Richard Chamberlain, but his character was compassionate and dedicated to his patients, and he understood them on a deep emotional level. I couldn't help being hooked on watching the adventures he became swept up in.

My old family doctor made house calls when family members were ailing in the early 1960s. All this combined to form my belief that doctors are infallible, benevolent, wise, and right next to God. After all, they healed and sustained our lives.

This set me up to trust that my primary care physician's magic elixirs and my surgeon's knife would heal me. My views quickly changed when I was diagnosed with CRPS and my doctors couldn't cure it and, in fact, sometimes made it worse—much worse.

Perhaps, like me, your current situation has changed your views about your health-care providers. In this chapter we'll delve into problems and solutions for accessing appropriate care. We'll explore the actions you can take so your health-care professionals will relate to you as a whole person rather than just a collection of symptoms. We'll also explore how telemedicine has transformed the relationship between health-care providers and patients. Finally, we'll address how to manage the advantages and stress of having immediate online access to test results.

As I've shared before, the injuries I sustained in my car accident in 1986 were devastating and forced me to search for help. My then-primary care physician was alarmed that his original prescription of rest didn't heal my body, and he referred me to an orthopedic surgeon for further treatment.

In the early days when Dr. Redhead, my orthopedist, couldn't nail down a diagnosis for me, he taught me that "Medicine is both an art and a science."

When he first said that, my eyes opened wide. The term "art" grabbed my attention. Art wasn't all-knowing. Art wasn't a guarantee. Art didn't increase my belief that he was going to improve my health. It lessened it. He was telling me that he didn't know everything. There were times the medical world was guessing!

Despite my dismay at learning he really wasn't God, I stayed with him. I liked him. I appreciated his honesty, and I felt I could trust him. After all, his guessing was better and more educated than my guessing. Maybe he could help my condition, even if he couldn't heal it. I chose to believe that he could make things better.

When, 24 months into my treatment, the anesthesiologist suggested I be evaluated for surgery at the prestigious medical school's pain clinic, I discussed it with Dr. Redhead. At that time, it wasn't widely recognized that surgery could spread CRPS. I accepted the required referral to the clinic, but unfortunately, as I shared in chapter 2, undergoing that surgery worsened my condition.

After my surgical fiasco, I returned to Dr. Redhead for ongoing care. He remained my treating physician until he retired 20 years later. Our relationship shifted, though. He understood that my surgery had further compromised my body, and he prescribed muscle relaxants and anti-inflammatory medications in the hope they would reduce my suffering.

He also encouraged me to explore complementary therapies like acupuncture, biofeedback, and massage because opioids weren't prescribed for chronic pain in the 1980s and the 1990s. Unfortunately, none of these complementary therapies (nonmainstream approaches) were covered by my insurance, so I had a lot of out-of-pocket expenses.

I also looked forward to discussing my forays into healing strategies that didn't have a price tag, like progressive relaxation and breathing exercises. Dr. Redhead would listen intently and ask questions, and he used my positive feedback as the basis to suggest mindfulness strategies to his other pain patients, who also found positive results.

Another thing that made him an exceptional doctor was that he maintained an accurate record of my condition and meticulously documented my case as required by the long-term disability insurance company. Many people who don't have doctors who stay on top of documenting disability information end up grappling with nerve-racking uncertainty around receiving disability benefits. Such oversights can cruelly halt or completely sever these crucial benefits, heaping yet another burden onto already anxious patients.

Over the decades since my diagnosis, I've had plenty of time to search for other health-care specialists to use in conjunction with my orthopedist. One thing was noticeably clear in this search: medical help is expensive. On top of that, a lot of pain patients experience extreme physical limitations. That results in 74% of them becoming unemployed and leads to those with severe pain spending $7,726 more annually on health-care costs than other patients.[124]

When I built my healing team, I tried to select professionals who were in my health maintenance organization's network to reduce my out-of-pocket expenses.

The most positive interactions I experienced with physicians and physical and occupational therapists were when they combined the science and art of their professions. They often asked questions about how my condition was impacting my life as a wife and mother. I always shared that my health created stress in my marriage. My then-husband loved to travel. Every few months, he enthusiastically combined a family vacation with a business trip. I would try to sound excited as I listened to him describe the latest greatest adventure he was planning for us, but in reality, I would be filled with dread.

I would be busy anticipating the agony I'd experience sitting on a plane or in a car for more than 30 minutes. Upon hearing my latest travel plans, some of my caring health-care professionals would provide suggestions like getting a neck pillow or an inflatable lumbar pillow to use on the plane and in the car, or packing an ice bag that could readily be filled from hotels' ice machines to quiet down my aching muscles.

---

124 "The Financial and Emotional Cost of Chronic Pain," U.S. Pain Foundation, September 29, 2021, https://uspainfoundation.org/news/the-financial-and-emotional-cost-of-chronic-pain/.

The practitioners who relied solely on the craft of their trade ignored the fact that I had a life beyond my diagnosis. They became frustrated when my health didn't improve. Some of them blamed my previous doctors who had treated me during the early days.

"I can't believe you let him do surgery on you," one of them exclaimed when his prescriptions didn't alleviate the symptoms that had been aggravated by my surgery.

Still others blamed me when their treatments failed. Even though I followed all their dietary suggestions, attended grueling early morning water therapy sessions, and always performed range of motion exercises, they implied that I wasn't trying hard enough when I didn't improve.

If I had to miss a therapy appointment to attend my son's school event or was required to go on a trip with my husband, they complained I wasn't giving 100% of my effort to heal. Some even believed I didn't have an incentive to improve because I was on long-term disability.

I have since heard from other patients that they were accused of making up their health issues, told that it was all in their head. Others had their doctors blame them for having too much stress in their lives. One doctor went so far as to tell a patient she'd heal if she lived on a beach in complete solitude.

The professionals who hinted that I wasn't in as much pain as I was telling them lost my business. Sometimes I would shake in anger at their arrogance to suggest that my lack of improvement was my fault. They had no idea how hard I was trying to get better.

Those doctors were overlooking the fact that, at that time, there were no known treatment approaches to help put CRPS into remission, and the best patients could hope for was a reduction in pain. So if doctors couldn't help my situation, I moved on to find those who I could cocreate a positive health-care experience with and who could help me minimize my symptoms.

What I was doing was building the right health-care team for me. It's your job to do that for yourself too. Equip yourself to stand firm against professionals who fault you for your condition or leave you doubting their expertise. Seek out those who have insight, skills, and the ability to guide you in your journey to improved health. If you haven't found them yet, don't lose heart; they exist. Sometimes finding them requires persistence.

Many factors will be at play as you create your treatment team. If you have health-care insurance, your first contact may have to be with a primary care physician. These physicians function as gatekeepers to specialists and other medical services like physical and occupational therapy. It's from primary care physicians that you'll receive referrals for further treatment. Sometimes these referrals may not be covered by your health plan, and you will incur out-of-pocket expenses.

Skyrocketing premiums, deductibles, and co-pays cause many people like me to navigate through their health plans' cost-covered treatment modalities before following through on the referrals they receive that require additional out-of-pocket expenditures. Others don't trust the mainstream system and would prefer alternative methods.

Still others are among the 30 million Americans without the safety net of health insurance.[125] Those plagued by chronic pain are wrestling with finances and grappling with how to pay for crucial medications and surgeries.

Another factor besides cost that can impact your choice of health-care professional is if your condition is a result of a work-related accident. Navigating the labyrinth of workers' comp can be challenging and overwhelming. Once

---

125   Nathan Paulus, "How Many Americans Are Uninsured?" Money Geek, last updated May 1, 2023, https://www.moneygeek.com/insurance/health/analysis/americans-without-coverage/.

a claim is lodged, it's typically your insurance carrier that selects your treating physician. The treatment is heavily influenced by the nature and longevity of your benefits. Your assigned representative can be critical to helping you through the process. But what's most important is for you to stay on top of things and be a fierce advocate for yourself and your health.

Even though I managed to connect with health-care providers who were covered by my insurance, as I mentioned earlier, many of the helpful complementary therapies were not covered, so over the decades, my treatment came at a hefty price.

I'm providing a list of the types of health-care providers I saw and the different therapies I explored during my 30-year journey to recover my health. You may be surprised not to see your type of specialist or therapy on my list. My selection was based on professionals who were comfortable treating my neurological condition, which was unusually perplexing due to my surgery. Some professionals I approached told me they couldn't do anything for me.

Acupuncturist

A trained practitioner inserts thin small needles into specific areas of the body to rebalance the body's energy flow and release blocked energy. This treatment activates the body's ability to heal emotionally, physically, and energetically. Acupuncture was helpful for my sciatica but didn't help my CRPS.

Many people find acupuncture helpful in treating back pain, joint pain, headaches, fibromyalgia, hormone imbalances, muscle spasms, and osteoarthritis.

This was an out-of-pocket expense for me.

Some but not all insurance plans cover acupuncture.

Anesthesiologist

The anesthesiologist I saw administered several types of nerve blocks that provided less than 36 hours of relief from my burning sensations. Many patients with back pain can obtain long-term relief from receiving an epidural nerve block. I wasn't one of them.

This was covered by my health insurance.

Aquatic Therapy

In aquatic therapy, a trained therapist helps the patient perform exercises in a heated pool for rehabilitation. This is good for neuromuscular and musculo-skeletal disorders. The buoyancy of the water reduces stress on the joints. This helped me regain the range of motion in my neck and my frozen shoulder.

This was an out-of-pocket expense for me.

It is possible to try aquatic therapy at a lower cost through Y programs that offer low to moderately priced group classes or through YouTube videos on water exercises that you can practice at your local public pool.

Biofeedback

This is a modality where a trained practitioner uses a biofeedback unit to help give patients greater awareness and control over physiological processes within their body. This unit consists of sensors and a monitor. The painless sensors are attached to various parts of a patient's body, and the patient is then instructed to observe results of their physiological changes on the monitor. These changes occur when they follow the practitioner's suggestions to alter breathing, change body positions, and concentrate on relaxing their muscles.

Viewing the changing numbers on the monitor teaches the patient that they can lessen their pain by changing the tension state in their body.

Tense muscles reduce the blood flow that carries nutrition and oxygen throughout the body, so they cause an increase in pain. Tense muscles also cause fatigue and soreness. To make matters worse, chronic tense muscles produce knots that dramatically increase suffering.

Biofeedback was always helpful for me during flare-ups. It gave me immediate feedback about the tension in my muscles. If there was a high level of tension, I then immediately concentrated on relaxing my muscles by deep breathing and using guided imagery to become more comfortable.

This was an out-of-pocket expense for me.

There are at-home units the size of a phone available that include sensors and a monitor. If you attach sensors to your body, the feedback will teach you to relax your muscles, which is important during a flare-up. These at-home units are in the $50+ range.

Dentist

My dentist created a custom night guard to help alleviate temporomandibular joint pain (TMJ) resulting from my neck injury. In some states, a visit to the orthodontist is required to be fitted for a guard. My dentist raised my awareness that the opioids and other medications I took were drying out my mouth. If that lasted too long, it would lead to extreme decay. She provided me with a protocol to maintain my dental health that involved not only brushing, using a Waterpik, and flossing, but also sucking on sugar-free moisturizing lozenges every three hours to add moisture to my mouth.

This was a partial out-of-pocket expense for me.

Dental insurance often covers part of the cost of a night guard. If your medications dry out your mouth, there are moisturizing lozenges and mouthwashes available over the counter that will protect your dental health.

Bilateral Music

A form of sound therapy that involves listening to music through headphones. The music is edited to consistently shift different tones to the right and left side of your headphones. These alternating tones have a soothing effect on the body because the music calms the regions of the brain that are prone to become more active when experiencing distressing events like a flare-up. Bilateral music is also useful for anxiety, stress, and trauma.

Whenever I listen to bilateral music, my relaxation response is stimulated as my brain balances the dual stimulation of the tones. It was my most effective tool when I was living with the stress of a flare-up.

This was an out-of-pocket expense for me during the 1990s before YouTube. Now there are freely available bilateral music videos on YouTube with comforting rhythmic music that relaxes the body and reduces pain.

Bodywork

These trained professionals manipulate the body's soft tissue, energy field, or both, which helps with stress and pain. There are many diverse types of bodywork, including neuromuscular therapy, polarity therapy, Reiki therapy, reflexology, sports massage, and Swedish massage.

I found massage therapy to be comforting rather than curative for my condition. Others have found it extremely helpful in giving them mobility and breaking down scar tissue buildup that causes pain. Massage also stimulates the lymphatic system, which reduces edema (accumulation of excess fluid in the tissues), removes waste and toxins from the body, and improves overall lymphatic drainage to enhance the body's immune response.

This was an out-of-pocket expense for me.

Bodywork is not usually covered by health-care insurance unless the therapist is affiliated with a chiropractic office.

Occupational Therapy

Therapists are trained in science-based methods to help patients improve their motor skills and their ability to perform daily living tasks. Occupational therapists come up with practical solutions to get things done, no matter your physical limitations.

My therapist taught me how to function in the kitchen and perform other daily living activities without the use of my dominant hand.

My occupational therapy was covered by my health insurance.

Orthopedist

Orthopedists are doctors who specialize in the musculoskeletal system. My orthopedist diagnosed my CRPS, prescribed medications, and documented my myofascial trigger points. For us nondoctors, myofascial trigger points are the tight bands of skeletal muscles inside a muscle group. Trigger points are tender when you touch them and can radiate pain to distant regions of the body. The physical therapists were able to apply effective deep tissue massage therapies for pain reduction through trigger point diagnosis.

These appointments were covered by my health insurance.

Physical Therapy

Trained therapists help patients improve and regain mobility, movement, flexibility, strength, balance, and coordination. They use manual techniques such as heat, cold, ultrasound, and electrical stimulation to reduce swelling and discomfort.

They treated my ongoing trigger points in my shoulder area and taught me to experiment with the settings of my TENS unit to relieve my flare-ups.

When I purchased my TENS unit in 1986, it required a prescription and was a $500 out-of-pocket expense. You can now buy a unit without a prescription for as little as $39 through Amazon.

My physical therapy was covered by my health insurance.

Primary Care Physician

This is often the main physician people see before going to a specialist. My current primary care physician prescribed pain medications in the past, but now that I'm off all pain-related medications, I continue to be seen for annual checkups.

These visits are covered by my health insurance.

Your list of health-care professionals may look different from mine because there are many different types of professionals who treat many types of chronic pain.

Your current or future team may include a professional from this list:

- **Chiropractor:** Practitioners who diagnose and treat neuromuscular disorders, most often by manually adjusting the spine, manipulating it, or both.[126] This helps upper and lower back pain and also pain in the hips, knees, and ankles. Chiropractors also focus on encouraging the body to heal itself.

- **Functional MD:** A conventionally trained MD who has decided to take an integrative approach to treat patients holistically. They obtain further training in order to find root causes of complex conditions that aren't easily resolved.

Rather than treating symptoms and diseases the way that a conventional MD does, they focus on the root cause of a disease/condition by analyzing a patient's environment, genetics, and biochemical and lifestyle factors. After reviewing the information and lab results, they create a multifaceted plan to treat the various causes of the condition.

Some of my clients who have extremely complex conditions have found great success through working with these doctors. When the doctor was able to determine several root causes of their health problems, the patients experience rapid improvement.

Tests associated with this type of treatment can come with a high price tag.

- **Naturopathic Doctor (ND):** This kind of doctor focuses on nutrition, homeopathic medicine, botanical medicine, hydrotherapy, stress management techniques, and other natural remedies. Their education can vary widely. Most focus on chronic pain, chronic fatigue, allergies, and hormone imbalances.

- **Doctor of Osteopathy (DO):** A DO focuses on treating the whole person by combining traditional medicine and osteopathic manip-

---

126 Steven Yeomans, "What Is a Chiropractor?" Spine-Health, March 14, 2013, https://www.spine-health.com/treatment/chiropractic/what-a-chiropractor.

ulative medicine. This manipulative medicine includes osteopathic manipulative technique (OMT). This is a hands-on noninvasive technique that involves applying gentle pressure to manipulate the body's muscles, joints, and tissues. It can reduce musculoskeletal pain, improve the patient's overall comfort, and, in some cases, reduce or replace the need for drugs or surgery. Osteopaths attend four years of medical school followed by residency training in their chosen specialty. They can prescribe medicine and perform surgeries.

- **Psychologist:** Some psychologists specialize in behavioral and emotional issues that accompany chronic pain. In searching for a psychologist, make sure that your psychologist has been trained in mind-body therapies.

- **Rheumatologist:** A conventional doctor who treats rheumatic diseases that cause pain, swelling, and stiffness in the bones, muscles, and joints, as well as other immune-related diseases. These diseases include gout, osteoarthritis, rheumatoid arthritis, lupus, and tendinitis.

Other options to receive health care to manage your chronic pain can include urgent care centers (also known as walk-in clinics), community health centers, online doctors, or teaching hospitals.

Whatever professional you're considering adding to your team, remember that communication is important in your health-care professional and patient relationship. You should have a voice in your treatment process. Studies show that when patients are engaged in a collaborative relationship, one where the professional and patient are seen as partners in the healing process, the patient experiences increased patient satisfaction and enhanced opportunity for a positive treatment outcome.[127]

These are the traits my best health-care providers demonstrated during office visits:

- Always communicated medical information in easy-to-understand language.

- Reviewed my chart before engaging with me.

- Questioned me about how my pain impacted all areas of my life.

- Listened to my successes and challenges with the most recent treatment protocols.

- Disengaged from the computer and maintained eye contact during our conversations.

- Respected my commitment to overcoming my chronic pain by providing appropriate referrals upon request.

- Responded in a timely manner to my phone calls and emails.

- When possible, provided me with samples of medications that I could try before they wrote me prescriptions not covered by my health plan.

- Accurately completed all required disability forms in a timely manner.

- Informed me of new treatments on the horizon.

- Gave me guidance and a choice about my treatment options.

- Respected my decisions when it came to my own health.

My collaborative relationships required that I attend every appointment

---

127   Sara Heath, "Good Patient-Provider Relationship Proves to Boost Outcomes," Xtelligent Healthcare Media, September 16, 2020, https://patientengagementhit.com/news/good-patient-provider-relationship-proves-to-boost-outcomes.

with an organized list of concerns and goals. I understood that it was vital to provide accurate information about my pain.

This list can help you provide information to your health professional:

- How long you've had your pain.

- Location of the pain—one region or all over?

- If pain is constant or intermittent.

- Duration of your pain.

- What actions increase or decrease the pain.

- Ways the pain limits your life.

- What triggers your pain.

When I had to describe my pain, I learned the adjectives I used could provide clues about the origin of my pain.

Here are some words that may apply to your pain:

- Aching
- Burning
- Cramping
- Dull
- Electrical shocks
- Freezing
- Gnawing
- Gripping
- Heavy
- Hot

- Numb
- Pounding
- Prickly
- Sharp
- Shooting
- Splitting
- Stabbing
- Tender
- Throbbing
- Visual disturbances with pain

If you have a hard time processing treatment information during your office visits, consider bringing a family member or friend to your appointments to take notes on your behalf. If you're concerned about sharing private information in front of them, have them stay in the waiting room until the doctor discusses the suggested treatment protocol.

Telemedicine

In March 2020, due to the pandemic, most of the world discovered that there was another way to meet with our doctors rather than traveling to the clinic. With the reduced regulations on telemedicine, we learned that our phones, tablets, and computers could be the gateway to consult with our health professionals from the comfort of our homes.

The terms "telehealth" and "telemedicine" filled the evening news as reporters covered stories of patients receiving care from the safety of their homes. Telehealth differs from telemedicine because it refers to a broader scope of remote health care than telemedicine.

"Telemedicine" refers specifically to remote clinical services that focus on diagnosis and treatment.

"Telehealth" not only includes remote clinical services but also medical education and training for medical professionals in the field. It's also a format for health system administrative meetings.[128]

My first telemedicine appointment in 2020 took place as I sat in my living room. I waited for my doctor to appear on the screen for my space-age house call. I was comfortable during my first virtual visit, and I continue to use telemedicine appointments and only book in-person appointments when it's

---

128 "Frequently Asked Questions," HealthIT.gov, accessed March 13, 2024, https://www.healthit.gov/faq/what-telehealth-how-telehealth-different-telemedicine.

time for my annual lab work and mammogram.

The public's overall acceptance of telemedicine during the pandemic motivated more health providers to add telemedicine to their practices. Doctors and mental health professionals were now eligible to be licensed to provide virtual care in states beyond their primary location.

If your health provider isn't set up for telemedicine, or if you're looking for a new doctor and want to try telemedicine, you can surf the internet to find scores of telemedicine doctors who offer appointments on demand. They can treat complaints including colds, flu, skin conditions, migraines, pain, allergies, and mental health issues, and they can provide prescription management. They can also review lab results, manage chronic health conditions, and order lab tests and scans. Their websites list the duration and price of a basic consultation.

The benefits of telemedicine include:

- No exposure to sick individuals as you sit in the waiting room.

- More convenient scheduling opportunities.

- Lower costs.

- Medical access for people without medical insurance.

- Medical access for people in rural areas.

- Medical access for people in underserved urban areas.

- Middle-of-the-night medical advice for babies and children.

- Limited need for childcare.

- Support for people with chronic illnesses who require frequent check-in appointments to access their ongoing health status.

- Online mental health care.

- Online physical therapy.

- No hassle of parking or use of any transportation.

- Easier to schedule around your work schedule.

Currently, the disadvantages of telemedicine include:

- Doctors can't use a stethoscope to listen to your heart or take vital signs.

- Visual assessments are more difficult to perform through a computer screen.

- It's not a substitute for emergency situations. It's important to head to the nearest hospital room if you're experiencing a crisis situation. Sometimes it can be hard to know if something is a crisis situation, and delays in receiving medical treatment can pose increased risk.

- Insurance coverage or reimbursement for telemedicine varies from state to state.[129]

Here are tips to prepare to use telemedicine:

- Plan ahead and write things down to refer to during your visit to ensure you'll have the information necessary to help your doctor understand your current health status.

- Make sure you have a reliable broadband or cellular connection for your phone, tablet, or computer.

- Check with your insurer about coverage and co-pays.

- Before the call, write down your symptoms and how long each one has been present.

---

129 Corey Whelan, "17 Benefits of Telemedicine for Doctors and Patients," Healthline, November 9, 2020, http://www.healthline.com/health/healthcare-provider/telemedicine-benefits.

- If you've had a fever, note the highs and lows and the duration.

- Have the medications and supplements you are taking for your current complaint available.

- List your preexisting conditions and any recent changes in your health.

- List any home care measures you have taken and their effectiveness.

- If you have a thermometer, blood pressure monitor, glucometer (for measuring sugar levels), and bathroom scale, have them available in case your provider requests a current reading.

- Find a quiet spot for your telemedicine appointment. Use earbuds or headphones to reduce outside noise during your videoconference and to ensure your privacy.

21st Century Cures Act

Telehealth and telemedicine aren't the only radical changes in health-care delivery that evolved in recent years. On December 13, 2016, the 21st Century Cures Act was passed, which required health providers to give patients immediate access to all their personal health information by April 5, 2021. This means patients can now view their past and present lab and imaging results, as well as their doctor's notes, online. Psychotherapy notes are excluded from being made available.[130]

Some patients feel empowered by being able to have immediate access to these reports. They're comfortable poring through their results and checking through the notes on their past office visits. Patients often search medical terms online when they see them in the reports and are motivated to expand their knowledge of medical terminology to decipher what the reports mean

---

130 Jen Tota McGivney, "Open Medical Records: Pros and Cons," Cancer Today, July 28, 2021, https://www.cancertodaymag.org/cancer-talk/open-medical-records-pros-and-cons/.

and not have to wait for their doctors to tell them.

One of the vexing outcomes of the 21ˢᵗ Century Cures Act, though, is that many patients lack the knowledge to be able to accurately interpret the reports. Many are troubled and confused by what they read. Online resources often don't provide them with an accurate understanding of the results. It's easy to make wrong conclusions and experience unnecessary panic without having a trained professional interpret the findings.

If you're uneasy about viewing your medical information, here are some tips:

- Refrain from reviewing results on a Friday afternoon since you'll have difficulty connecting with your provider if you have questions about your report.

- Most importantly, if you find that reviewing your results is disturbing, wait to view them until your doctor can explain the findings.

Case Study: Diabetic Peripheral Neuropathy

The previous case studies I've presented are clients who reached out to me for help. This case study involves the landscape architect/auto mechanic/stand-up comedian I first mentioned in chapter 8. We formed a strong bond when he helped me create my thriving perennial garden. I became his go-to health coach after helping him overcome back spasms he had complained about when we first met. Eventually we fell into a pattern where we'd meet at our local wholesale nursery every time he had a health concern. He educated me about plants as I provided health education about his latest challenge.

Diabetic Peripheral Neuropathy

Diabetic peripheral neuropathy is a common destructive result of long-term high blood sugar levels from type 1 and type 2 diabetes. It most often affects the legs and feet and sometimes the arms and hands. The excess levels of sugar injure the walls of the capillaries (tiny blood vessels that nourish the nerves). This causes nerve damage to the circulatory network. This damage interferes with the transmissions of sensory messages between the central nervous system (brain and spinal cord) and all other parts of the body.[131]

People of all ages with type 1 and type 2 diabetes are fair game for developing this additional condition.

Symptoms of peripheral neuropathy can cause people to disregard an injury or a lesion on the foot because numbness in their limb prevents them from feeling the wound. Also, poor circulation caused by diabetes can hinder wound healing. This increases the risk of infection. In the most extreme cases, a chronic wound can lead to amputation.

Patients sometimes experience symptoms more frequently in the evening.

Symptoms

- Numbness

- Burning or tingling sensations

- Extreme sensitivity to touch

- Muscle weakness

- Loss of coordination and balance

---

131 Carmella Wint, Matthew Solan, and Brian Wu, "Everything You Should Know About Diabetic Neuropathy," Healthline, November 22, 2022, https://www.healthline.com/health/type-2-diabetes/diabetic-neuropathy.

- Serious foot problems including ulcers, infections, and bone and joint damage

- Erectile dysfunction

Risk Factors

- High blood sugar levels over a long period of time

- Damage to blood vessels due to high cholesterol levels

- Mechanical injury such as carpal tunnel syndrome

- Lifestyle factors such as smoking or alcohol consumption

- Low levels of vitamin B12

Diagnosis

- Case history of symptoms

- Physical examination

- Lab work

- Sensory tests

Treatments

- Anticonvulsant medications

- Antidepressant medications

- Capsaicin cream (pepper derivative that helps nerve pain)

- TENS unit

- Acupuncture

- Prevent further progression of the condition

- Monitor blood glucose levels

- Take medications as prescribed

- Avoid smoking

- Avoid alcohol

- Maintain an exercise program

- Avoid foods with added sugar and saturated and trans fats

- Adhere to a heart-friendly diet

On a foggy Monday morning in May, I drove the back roads of San Ramon, California, heading to my favorite wholesale nursery. On this unseasonably cold spring day, I wore hiking boots, black jeans, a black pullover sweater, and my warm REI jacket. I was looking forward to meeting up with Hugo, one of my most humorous clients.

As I pulled onto the nursery's unpaved parking lot, I wondered what health issue I'd be hearing about that morning. The place was crowded with gardeners who were loading plants and fertilizer onto the beds of their trucks. I got out of the car, zipped up my jacket, and heard, "Hey, Chaplain Bonnie!" I turned and saw Hugo standing in between a row of Japanese maples and crepe myrtle trees.

At 6'4" he was taller than the trees. His wavy auburn hair was shorter than I remembered; he used to wear it in a ponytail, but now it was about chin length. He was only 42 years old, but his thick beard and handlebar mustache showed hints of gray. He had a low cart right next to him and bent to place a crepe myrtle sapling onto it. The sleeves of his sweatshirt were pushed up, revealing his muscular forearms that were covered with flower and parrot tattoos.

"I didn't see your green work truck," I called out as I hurried over to him.

He pointed to an apple-red vintage 1953 Ford F-100. I'd forgotten that he loved to restore vintage trucks. What I hadn't forgotten was that the last time we had walked among the plants, he had been reeling from a diagnosis of type 2 diabetes. He rarely got sick and didn't believe in regular medical checkups. The diabetes was discovered when he applied for additional life insurance after he married his soulmate.

I'd received a frantic call after he had learned he had to give himself daily injections of insulin. He had a phobia of shots and didn't want to tell his doctor. He had asked if I could help him overcome his phobia. We met through Zoom the next day, and I guided him to envision himself holding a hypodermic and feeling calm. His shoulders immediately eased, and his breathing slowed. He concentrated on keeping his muscles relaxed. When he learned the breathing technique, he moved on to actually holding the hypo-dermic. He practiced filling the syringe with water and injecting an orange, keeping his muscles relaxed as he did so.

When he shifted to injecting himself with insulin, he was able to stay calm, but when he smelled the alcohol to sterilize the injection site, he got stressed. I suggested he douse a cotton ball with his favorite pine essential oil and place it nearby. Inhaling its scent while thinking about his current truck restoration project as he inserted the needle into his skin would override the triggering smell of alcohol. I couldn't wait to find out how that had gone.

We walked toward a display of red-and-white lipstick salvia plants that never failed to attract hummingbirds.

"How are you doing with your insulin shots?" I asked.

He finished placing six perennial salvias on the cart.

"Piece of cake. Used the same visualization techniques when I got my tetanus shot."

"That's great to hear."

The sapling and the salvias wobbled as he pulled the cart over the gravel, heading off toward the succulent tent. The fog had burned off, and it looked like it was going to be a warm day.

"My feet feel like they're asleep, though, and I have sensations like pins and needles poking into my calves."

So that was his latest health issue.

"What'd your doctor say?"

"I'm too busy. The housing market is going nuts, and all the real estate agents are calling me to 'pretty up' their clients' yards so they can get the houses on the market," he continued. "I'll lose a half day of work if I go to see my doctor."

I was glad to hear his business was thriving, but the symptoms he was describing sounded like diabetic peripheral neuropathy. That's a common problem for diabetics, and it's serious.

We entered the tent, and I saw a vast collection of orange, green, and red plants. I bent over to read the names and descriptions, reached for a vibrant green agave plant, and placed it on the cart.

"You've got to be careful of that agave species because it has a prickly sticker at the tip of the leaves. I don't want your grandkids to get pricked and get an infection." He returned it to the shelf and replaced my selection with a beautiful green-and-crimson jade plant.

I stared at his replacement plant, which was going to make a great addition to my backyard, then back up at him. "Thank you for that."

We strolled several feet before I said, "It's important to connect with your doctor."

"My A1C is doing good," he blurted out. Then, as an afterthought, he added, "I'm following the diabetic dietary guidelines most of the time."

Every diabetic I know can recite their A1C results. This simple blood test measures the blood sugar levels for the past three months. Monitoring A1C is an important tool in managing diabetes.

"That's good news, but it's important that you tell your doctor about the sensations you're experiencing."

We stopped walking and stared at the velvet-like kangaroo paw plants. Their bright orange color was vibrant and popped.

"You could do a video appointment with your doctor from your work or your home."

He looked over at me reluctantly. "I didn't think of that."

"You really shouldn't put it off."

He frowned.

"Why don't we meet on Zoom tonight to prepare a list of your symptoms and questions for the doctor to help you feel organized for your telemedicine appointment?"

That night on our call, behind him I saw a large black-and-white tuxedo cat lounging on top of a bookshelf filled with small cactus plants. I also heard the familiar squawking of the Amazon parrot he had adopted from my flock.

My goal that night was to teach him the importance of sharing his symptoms with his doctor.

After a brief greeting, I started the session by asking, "When you get a call from somebody whose vintage truck needs to be fixed, do you ask them all about the problem?"

"Sure," he said.

"The more information you get, the easier it is to find a solution."

"True," he said.

"Think of your body like a truck and your doctor like the mechanic. You've got to help your doctor understand what's going on."

I used a diabetic neuropathy symptom checklist I had downloaded from a diabetic information website to ask about his current symptoms. When we got to erectile dysfunction (ED), a quite common diabetic neuropathy symptom in men, he shifted uncomfortably in his chair and then cracked a joke.

"What do waterfalls take when they have erectile dysfunction?…Niagara."

"There are ED medications your doctor could prescribe," I said, avoiding his diversion.

"Yeah, I see ads for them on TV all the time, so I guess a lot of other guys are having the same problem."

We had a follow-up Zoom meeting two weeks after he had his telemedicine meeting. This time, I saw that the bookcase behind him was full of seedling containers with LED grow lamps positioned in front of them.

"I've got early symptoms of diabetic peripheral neuropathy," he said glumly. "The doc prescribed medication to cut down on the irritating sensations. He said the food plan I'm on will help, but I need to cut out bad fats and add flax, hemp, and chia seeds to help reduce my neuropathy."

"Those ingredients are easy to add to your meals, and an added plus is that they contribute to eye health."

"There's some good news to share. It turns out that the strenuous exercise I get from my work will slow down the progression of the nerve damage."

"That is good news." I smiled at him, thinking how young he was to be suffering nerve damage. I knew all too well how hard that could be. "How was it meeting with your doctor?"

A slow smile crossed his face. "I like the convenience of telemedicine. When I scheduled the appointment, I even went into my online patient chart for the first time and saw my lab work."

"Did you feel stressed out to view your lab numbers?"

"Seeing the original lab work from when I was first diagnosed blew my mind because my A1C number was so high, but now I'm doing great."

"Did you share *everything* on your list?" I raised my eyebrows, hoping he knew what I was talking about.

He immediately looked sheepish. "He prescribed little blue pills to help my romantic situation." Looking away from the camera, he added, "The pills give me a stomachache, so I'm not using them."

"There might be other ED pills he can prescribe. But in the meantime, why don't you learn more about improving your circulatory health? That might also help the situation. In fact, you might want to read *Prevent and Reverse Heart Disease* by Caldwell B. Esselstyn, Jr. That talks about how diet can heal arteries and improve circulatory issues. You can also watch his YouTube interviews, where he talks about eating a small serving of greens six times a day to improve neuropathy and to help solve ED issues."[132]

As the months passed, Hugo's landscape work kept him so busy that he increased the size of his usual crew. Whenever he had extra plants from projects in my town, Dublin, I'd come home and find them sitting on my front porch with a simple smiley face sticky note attached.

I was always thrilled to receive another plant for my garden, and I used my thank-you texts as an opportunity to ask how he was doing. This was always our ongoing check-in pattern until one day, out of the blue, he initiated a check-in by sending a happy text telling me his uncomfortable neuropathy sensations were completely controlled by his dietary changes and medication. He added that eating greens six times a day had solved his "romantic problem," so he no longer needed ED medication, and his new bride was thrilled.

In this chapter, just like Hugo, you learned the importance of establishing a collaborative relationship with your health professionals. Whether your physician is a mainstream physician (MD), an osteopath (DO), a functional doctor, or a holistic practitioner, the relationship you establish can influence your treatment outcome.

We also explored how to best assist your doctor to accurately diagnose your condition and develop an effective pain treatment plan by presenting an accurate description of your pain and what activates or calms it.

Finally, you learned that telemedicine and the 21st Century Cures Act have put you in the driver's seat of your health. You can now experience a medical appointment in your home and have your past medical notes and lab reports available during your appointment.

---

132 Esselstyn, *Prevent and Reverse Heart Disease.*

In the next chapter, you'll have the opportunity to create your personalized plan of action to reduce your suffering. By the time you complete the chapter, you'll be empowered to achieve living a life in control of your pain.

▍ REMEMBER:

- There's a wide range of health providers who treat chronic pain.

- A positive relationship with your health-care provider can improve treatment outcomes.

- Descriptive pain words are an important tool for doctors to understand the origin of your pain.

- Telemedicine offers a cost-reducing option for timely medical care.

- The 21st Century Cures Act enables you to access your medical notes, lab results, and scan reports.

CHAPTER 16

All About You

♥

"Take good care of your body. It's the only place you have to live."
—JIM ROHN, AUTHOR AND MOTIVATIONAL SPEAKER

Congratulations! We've gone on quite a journey, uncovering affordable and accessible effective tools to reduce our pain and increase our vitality. I hope you're as excited as I am that your chronic pain doesn't have to be a life sentence.

Through the power of applying the concept of neuroplasticity and working with the nervous system, we discovered that we could rewire our experience of pain to lessen or eliminate it completely. We also found out that, through incorporating positive changes in our lifestyle behaviors, we can improve our overall health. And finally, through the power of taking our health in our own hands, we learned that self-care could make an enormous difference in our overall quality of life.

We watched other pain patients like you use simple techniques and achieve remarkable results.

To help you quickly remember as you take steps to the new you, here's a recap of the key principles:

- The pain loops that we are currently experiencing can be changed by doing a customized homemade retraining program (chapter 1).

- How it's possible to redefine yourself despite your pain (chapter 2).

- How the AIM (Affirmation, Image, and Management) program helps us to reclaim an identity beyond being a pain sufferer (chapter 3).

- What pain is and why we experience it (chapter 4).

- The differences between acute and chronic pain, and how we can diminish our suffering (chapter 4).

- The four foundational strategies we can use to reduce pain today (chapter 5).

- The benefits of self-care (chapter 6).

- The best pain management system (chapter 7).

- How to retrain our brains to be less reactive, experience less trauma, and, overall, to reduce our symptoms (chapter 7).

- The impact our environment has on our condition and how humor can help (chapter 8).

- The life-sustaining fuel nutritious food gives us in our recovery (chapter 9).

- How to know which foods are most supportive for our overall health (chapter 9).

- The power of incorporating gentle movement into our daily life and how movement aids our muscles to relax and improves our mood (chapter 10).

- The substances that are destroying our health and increasing our pain—and what to do about them (chapter 11).

- The physiological and psychological impact of stress on the body's systems and what to do to reduce its impact (chapter 12).

- How to boost the quality of our sleep to increase our body's healing capability (chapter 13).

- How to stop isolation in its tracks even when chronic pain is at its peak (chapter 14).

- Steps to enhance our relationship with our health-care providers in order to work as a team (chapter 15).

- The different options for health care for those dealing with chronic conditions (chapter 15).

- Ways to participate in telemedicine care and access our online medical records (chapter 15).

Reviewing the list of everything we've learned to improve our situation might look overwhelming. Don't worry. Remember, the people highlighted in the case studies are individuals whose lives quickly improved after they implemented just a few of the strategies. The improvement they experienced lifted their spirits and bolstered their motivation to add in a few more strategies. The same thing can happen for you when you apply the most relevant suggestions.

Opening the Door to Change

Fourteen years ago, I was among the more than 50 million adults in America who suffered from chronic pain.[133] We all had the same wish—for the pain to end. I was able to remove myself from that statistic by applying the kernel of knowledge of neuroplasticity gleaned during my husband's scary ER visit as well as the foundational knowledge I'd learned decades before in my college courses on the precursor to today's lifestyle medicine.

Knowing that it was possible to change my brain launched me on my path, where I eventually learned that I had the power to become my own change agent. By taking active steps, trying out simple homemade neuroplasticity solutions, and using the six pillars of lifestyle medicine to guide me, I was able to dramatically reduce my suffering. I now have a life full of vitality and strength that has enabled me to bravely write a *very* personal book about my experience, just to inspire you to become your own change agent with your health.

Walking the Dog Changed Everything

Back in 2010 when I laced up my shoes to walk my neighbor's dog, I had no idea that the adventure I was embarking on would bring me to the place I am today, enjoying adventures, socializing with friends, and maintaining a busy pain coaching schedule. My decision to design my own brain experiments started with changing my 24-year pain habit of grimacing, clenching my teeth, wincing, and talking to myself about how bad I felt.

I put on a fake smile and, whenever I greeted another dog walker, I avoided engaging in any conversation about my health problems. For the first time since 1986, I was "acting as if" I was pain-free. Smiling actually improved my mood. Smiles stimulate the amygdala to release oxytocin, a happy neurotrans-

---

133   S. Michaela Rikard, "Chronic Pain Among Adults—United States, 2019–2021," *Morbidity and Mortality Weekly Report* 72, no. 15 (April 14, 2023), https://www.cdc.gov/mmwr/volumes/72/wr/pdfs/mm7215a1-H.pdf.

mitter.[134] (For us nonscientists, the amygdala is the part of our brain that processes memory, decision-making, and emotional responses.) I later learned that by vanquishing pain reactions, I created new neural pathways in my brain. These new pathways eventually made my brain perceive less pain, and thus I experienced less.

Make Self-Care Yours

Now that you've read the whole book and know your options, it's time to practice smiling in front of a mirror and think about how you can incorporate your self-care program into your life.

I found one of the best ways to approach this is to answer these questions:

- What will it look like when my condition improves?

- What can I do right now that would improve my health?

- What can I try that might reduce my pain?

- How can I customize my program so I'll stick to it?

If you aren't able to answer these questions yet, remember that some of the individuals I highlighted in my case studies didn't believe they could minimize their pain. They "acted as if" and kept that up until things got better.

Whether you are "all in" or using the "act as if" approach, the methods in this book are available to you day or night. You don't have to travel to a clinic or a gym. Also, you won't have to deplete your bank account to purchase costly equipment or services that may not be covered by your health insurance and may not work.

---

134 "When You're Smiling, the Whole World Really Does Smile with You," University of South Australia, August 12, 2020, https://www.unisa.edu.au/media-centre/Releases/2020/when-youre-smiling-the-whole-world-really-does-smile-with-you/.

Your Customized Homemade Program

I created a customization system called "ABOUT ME" to help you incorporate pain management hacks into your day-to-day life. Pain doesn't disappear overnight, nor does it dramatically diminish on a specific time schedule, but it can be reduced.

ABOUT ME is a system for you to develop your unique program to diminish your discomfort. It works by giving you seven different lenses through which to view your unique challenge. By guiding yourself through the many ways to approach your situation, you invite more insights to produce more creative solutions than would result if you looked at your problems in only one or two ways.

The guiding principle when working through the system is to remember that you're an experiment of one. What your body needs is unique to you.

Here's the overview of the system's seven lenses that will help you construct your personalized improvement programs.

ABOUT ME

1. **A = Approach:** This is the time to look at how you are viewing your discomfort and decide if there would be a better way to view it. *How can I improve my outlook about a challenge I want to undertake?*

2. **B = Behavior:** Pay attention to your current behaviors that might be contributing to the problem. *What am I doing that's adding to my suffering?*

3. **O = Observe:** Observe what is happening in your body and your environment that might be contributing to the problem. *How is my*

environment aggravating my condition?

4. **U = Understand:** Time to gain as much understanding as possible about why you are having the discomfort you are experiencing by studying what the research says to do to help the problem. *What proof is there in science/research that these behaviors will help?*

5. **T = Tools:** Look for any mind-body exercises or affordable and accessible devices that would make it easier for you to minimize your discomfort. *Which ideas and methods am I comfortable using and do I have access to?*

6. **M = Motivate:** When working with chronic pain, it's important to stay inspired to keep going when things become really tough. *What reward will make me feel I'm making progress and keep me showing up?*

7. **E = Educate:** Discover the best place to stay on top of the latest research and findings. *Where can I obtain further information and support?*

ABOUT ME in Action—Chaplain Bonnie's Personal ABOUT ME Program

To give you a better idea about how this system has served me and my clients for years, I want to tell you how I personally used it. I applied this program when I experienced a flare-up after I aggravated an old whiplash injury while I was in the process of authoring this book. The painful spasms I experienced got in the way of typing, driving a car, preparing meals, and my daily chore of cleaning my six parrot cages. I was frustrated and bummed out that my flare-up was interrupting my writing progress and all my other responsibilities.

Step 1: Approach

I thought about how I was approaching the situation—angry that my flare-up was interrupting my schedule. The more I thought about it, the more irritated I became. The anger was causing a negative emotional impact on me, so that had to change.

I played with affirmations until I found one that felt incredibly supportive: "I know this is a temporary inconvenience. I'll be able to do things to loosen up my neck to increase my range of motion. When my neck quiets down, I'll be able to resume my day-to-day activities."

Step 2: Behavior

I thought about all the activities I had been doing in the days and hours before my flare-up. The prior three days had been hectic. I had sat typing for hours without a break during the morning. In the afternoons, I had sat training clients through Zoom. When I had gotten a break between Zoom appointments, I had been busy chopping and dicing veggies and fruit for a week's worth of stews, soups, salads, and parrot meals.

Reviewing my behavior revealed I'd ignored the importance of getting in stretching activities before signing on to each new meeting. This flare-up taught me that my daily early morning aerobics weren't enough to prevent my shoulders and neck from aching. I needed to routinely take a break to stretch my neck and shoulders throughout the day.

Step 3: Observe

I played detective and studied my desk setup. To my surprise, my adjustable desk was set in a lower position than usual. My wireless keyboard was lying flat rather than sitting at the angle I usually use to reduce stress on my wrists.

I fixed everything to fit my body and its needs better. I wondered how this could have happened.

It took a day before I remembered that, a few weeks prior, I'd moved my computer so I could use my adjustable desk to work on a jewelry project that had required me to lower the desk and to move my keyboard off to the side.

Step 4: Understand

I was disappointed in myself for forgetting to take breaks to stretch my body. Additionally, I had neglected to maintain a comfortable office environment. This lack of attention had caused my neck and wrists to become strained, leading to the development of spasms that I could easily have avoided if I had paid attention.

The neck spasms had significantly disrupted my life. My basic chores were becoming a challenge, so I found myself needing assistance. The discomfort also made putting together PowerPoint presentations for my upcoming workshops a challenge.

As I watched myself beat myself up, I knew that I wasn't being kind to myself. I stopped the shamefest and resolved that I would pay more attention when I worked on other projects. It was now mandatory for me to restore my work environment before I began any of my computer activities.

Step 5: Tools

To manage my neck pain, I used a warm compress for 20 minutes every few hours. When my muscles felt comforted by the heat, I repeatedly shrugged my shoulders to relax my muscles and gently turned my head back and forth to loosen the muscles.

Once the tension in those muscles eased, my back muscles started shouting, wanting attention too. I whipped out my TENS unit to calm them. The pulses from the unit blocked the angry messages being generated by my brain.

I had to accept the simple fact that I couldn't maintain my usual schedule. My disciplined personality found that very irritating, but I knew it was best not to dwell on it. If my body needed rest and recovery, it was only going to scream louder until I gave in. Besides, it was my fault that I'd slipped into poor body mechanics.

I propped myself up with pillows to support my achy muscles and relaxed using deep breathing exercises while I listened to guided imagery tapes. I was surprised that I was relaxed enough to take a rare nap. My mood also improved when I made sure to take time to stimulate my feel-good neurotransmitters by having a pleasant conversation with a friend. I also spent time relaxing in my bird room and watching my parrots' antics.

Within 24 hours, the muscles in my neck calmed, but I was still uncomfortable. It was time to work on the trigger points in my shoulders. I've found my handheld massage wand helps relax and release my trigger points.

Step 6: Motivate

This flare-up taught me I needed a reminder to consistently perform the behaviors necessary to keep me at the top of my game. For motivation I decided to go wild and award myself purple paper clips every time I executed appropriate behavior to help prevent a flare-up. My growing purple paper clip chain hangs off my bulletin board in my office. The other motivational tool I use is setting my phone alarm to remind me to get up and stretch.

Step 7: Educate

I researched the latest ergonomic strategies for minimizing muscle strain while working at the computer. I learned that, by alternating sitting with standing while working at my computer, I could avoid future flare-ups. I also found a well-designed mouse that's easier to navigate with than the one I was using. And finally, I learned that using the Dictate tool in Word is a great alternative to typing.

What I learned from working through the system was that I could manage a pesky neck and shoulder flare-up and how to minimize the chance of it happening in the future.

My clients who used the system found that it helped them not only with their physical challenges but also with those instances when their emotions got the better of them. I had taught them how emotions amplify their discomfort (the same information I share in chapter 7). Applying the lenses of ABOUT ME helped them overcome despair, frustration, and lack of motivation. If you're willing to work through the steps, ABOUT ME can also work for you too.

In conclusion, I created the ABOUT ME system and all the other original ideas presented in this book during my three-decade struggle to overcome my pain syndrome. It was during that time that a doctor once asked me what I hoped to do if I ever got better. I said, "To make a difference in people's lives." My social media inspirational posts, the lifestyle medicine classes I teach through Zoom, and this book are a result of that long-ago desire.

I hope the time you've spent with me has inspired you to continue your healing journey.

HOPE = Hold On, Pain Ends

Wishing you strength, courage, and humor for today and all your tomorrows.

Chaplain Bonnie's Blessing for You

Appendix A

Bonus Case Study: Back Pain—The Universal Pain Experience

During the early days of the pandemic, a fretting wife reached out to me and begged me to meet with her borderline type 2 diabetic husband, Jeff, who had recently become chronically depressed due to an extremely uncomfortable protruding disc. She was alarmed that a blanket of gloom was descending over him, and he had recently lost interest in his passion for vintage cars.

On a chilly late September afternoon, a man with an abundant frame lumbered in my direction for our first walk session. His heavy work boots crunched the pile of orange-and-brown leaves. His dark sunglasses seemed to anchor his blue mask as his salt-and-pepper beard peeked out below the mask. I had prepared myself for this meeting by researching vintage cars because I knew that was his passion.

He stopped right in front of me and crossed his arms. "Are you Chaplain Bonnie?"

"Yes." I nodded. "You must be Jeff."

"Yeah. I've got a bad back."

Chronic Back Pain

In America, 16 million adults suffer from chronic back pain, making it a leading cause of work limitations and work-loss days.[135] If pain persists with the following symptoms, it's important to have your back checked out by a health-care professional such as an orthopedist, a chiropractor, or an osteopath.

Symptoms

- Pain after a fall or injury

- Weakness, pain, burning, or numbness in your legs

- Fever

- Difficulty urinating

Risk Factors[136]

- Muscle or ligament strain

- Bulging or ruptured disks

- Arthritis

- Osteoporosis

- Ankylosing spondylitis

Diagnosis

- Physical exam

---

135 "Chronic Back Pain," Health Policy Institute, accessed February 21, 2024, https://hpi.georgetown.edu/backpain/.

136 "Back Pain," Mayo Clinic, February 19, 2023. https://www.mayoclinic.org/diseases-conditions/back-pain/symptoms-causes/syc-20369906

- X-ray and scans if the condition merits it

- Depending on the findings, lab tests might be ordered to see if an infection is causing the issue

- Nerve studies if there is numbness, weakness, burning, or tingling present

Treatments

- Analgesics (acetaminophen, aspirin)

- Nonsteroidal anti-inflammatory drugs (ibuprofen, naproxen)

- Muscle relaxants

- Topical pain relievers

- Tricyclic antidepressants to reduce uncomfortable sensations

- Cortisone injections

- Radiofrequency ablation

- TENS unit

- Implanted nerve stimulators

- Surgery

At-Home Treatment

- Resting

- Staying hydrated

- Gentle massage

- Supportive mattress and pillows

- Ice for the first 48 hours to reduce inflammation, then switch to a heating pad to relax the muscles

- Over-the-counter pain relievers

- Gentle stretching exercises to improve flexibility and strength

- Maintaining good posture to reduce strain

Jeff suffered from a protruding disc in his lower spine. His doctor prescribed walking and strengthening exercises to stop spasms. Understanding the high risk of his situation, after our greeting, I launched in. "Are you ready to do what it takes to feel better now?"

He exhaled a heavy sigh. "I'm here."

We rounded the corner of the track as the sun glared straight into our eyes.

"My whole body aches so bad I can barely lift my legs to walk," he mumbled. "This is unbearable…" On and on he complained. "I'm doomed to a life of pain. It's in the family. Both my grandfather and father suffered with bad backs and type 2 diabetes. Give me a few years and I'll have full-blown type 2 diabetes and a worse back."

This had to stop, now.

I blurted out, "Tell me why, in 1936, did they make only four Bugatti Type 57 SC Atlantic sedans that are now worth millions of dollars?"

That question flipped the conversation right into a big spiel about cars. Jeff talked the whole way around the track two times without pausing for breath, telling me about the unique history of the sedans.

Out of breath from our fast clip around the track, I asked, "How're you feeling?"

He looked at me through his fogged-up glasses, surprised. "Good."

As soon as I saw that he was in a good mood at our next car talk/walk session, I went after him about increasing his fiber to help his body's production of mood enhancement hormones.

"Are you saying I have to diet?" Jeff immediately snapped.

"Nope. Eliminate highly processed foods like chips, bacon, and hotdogs and add vegetables and fruit. That way, you'll be creating a healthier relationship between your gut and your brain."

"That doesn't sound fun."

"Imagine you're at a busy airport with people crowding the hallways and others rushing as they run to catch their planes."

His walking had slowed, but at least he was listening. "Okay?"

"This busy activity in the airport is the 100 trillion microorganisms living in the gut zipping around doing their jobs. When the gut gets enough fiber, things go smoothly, like in a busy international airport on a good day. But if there are disturbances like plane cancelations and storms raging, or, in the gut's case, lack of fiber and nutritional support, things go into massive confusion quickly."

"I've experienced a crowded airport one Thanksgiving. It was a nightmare."

"I imagine." I was glad that I never got near an airport on a major holiday. "In order to keep our gut moving smoothly, we need to keep our microbiome happy." Our pace around the track had picked up.

"I've heard about that on the radio. It seems like it's really important."

"It is. It helps you digest food and supports your immune system, heart, and brain health. The strength of the microbes is influenced by the type of foods eaten. For example, when the microbiome consumes fiber, it'll secrete hormones that not only help your immune system and heart but can stabilize your weight."

"I get what you're telling me. I don't like it, but I get it." He was silent for at least 20 seconds before saying, "Small steps."

Now that I had his buy-in, it was time to make it easier for him. Making such dramatic dietary changes was no easy feat. "I want you to make a playlist of all your favorite songs and listen to them in the morning to put you in a good mood."

He pursed his lips. "Are you trying to make my wife happy?"

"Of course," I chuckled. "And I want you to listen to them when you're in pain, too, to shift your focus. Also, I'd like you to set up a daily schedule of activities that interest you."

The next check-in, he reported that the music thing was working, and his bathroom time had become more comfortable due to increased fiber. For the daily mood assignment, after listening to his favorite songs, he cheerfully watched short videos about restoring trucks.

I suggested that he award himself with a paper clip each time he added fiber to his meals and listened to his music. "I'd like to see a paper clip chain at least seven clips long the next time we meet."

"Gotcha," he said, "and your assignment is to research the 1951 Ford F-1."

Through October and into December, Jeff's chain hung in his living room to remind him he was moving toward a pain-free life. He consistently walked, did back exercises, used caution lifting his automotive tools, and enthusiastically did his mood-elevating activities. He changed from chips and a sour cream-based dip to raw vegetables dipped in hummus. He also reduced the amount of oil and sugar in his diet.

Before our last walk, he sent me two photos, one showing his long paper clip chains and one showing two leather belts. The first was the larger belt he had worn on the day we met. The smaller belt was the one he now uses to hold up his loosening slacks. Not only did the weight loss diminish the strain on his back, but he was also out of danger of developing type 2 diabetes. By Christmas, his chain spread from the ceiling halfway to the floor.

To complete my homework assignment, I learned that the 1951 Ford F-1 chassis, known as the prototype for the iconic "Beatnik Bandit" car, was the result of Ford's million-dollar research to increase cabin comfort. Designed by legendary Ed "Big Daddy" Roth, it was nicknamed the Million-Dollar Cab.

Overall, these simple assignments guided Jeff from suffering to a more active and fulfilling life. On our final walk, Jeff said he appreciated that all the self-care strategies I taught him were accessible 24/7. This helped him cope with a nighttime flare-up that occurred after he spent an afternoon lifting his grandkids onto swings at the park. He was also appreciative that whenever I suggested a useful pain management technique, he never had to rob a bank.

Postscript

Over the years, I have received hundreds of photos of paper clip chains from people who have incorporated my simple reward system into their self-care routines. If you have a box of paper clips in a drawer somewhere in your house, you're only one paper clip away from being well on your way to lowering your pain.

REMEMBER:

- Changing behavior leads to improved health.

- The mind-body approach is effective in reducing pain.

- Customizing behavioral strategies makes them easy to incorporate into your life.

- Reward systems increase motivation.

Appendix B

Hacks for a Flare-Up That's Got You Down

A flare-up is a sudden increased intensity of pain. It can be unpredictable and usually occurs without warning. The increased pain can be debilitating, both physically and emotionally.

There are many possible triggers for a flare-up:

- Stress

- Fatigue

- Weather changes

- Poor overall diet, including inflammatory foods and drinks like fried and processed food, sodas, gluten (for those sensitive), red wine, caffeine, dairy (for those sensitive), and red meat

- Hormonal changes

- Infection

- Overdoing physical activity such as housework, yard work,

and exercise

- Disruption in practicing effective treatment strategies

A flare-up can be intensified by a strong emotional response. If a person feels frustrated and angry about the flare-up, it will increase the distress. A great way to stop or lessen negative feelings is to have a solid plan for how to handle a flare-up.

Strategies to Handle a Flare-Up

- Remind yourself that this is just a temporary setback and that, by using self-care strategies, you'll be able to reduce your discomfort.[137]

- Change your schedule to accommodate self-care.

- If you have specific medications for a flare-up, take them as prescribed.

- Use pillows to support the uncomfortable parts of your body.

- Apply heat, ice, or a combination of both if it quiets down your pain and is recommended by your doctor.

- A moist heat compress can be created by filling an athletic sock with rice and tying it off with a knot. Heat in the microwave on high for two minutes.

- A frozen bag of corn or peas can be used as an ice pack.

- Use a handheld massage wand to relax major muscle groups to release the tension.

- Take a warm shower or soak in a warm bath with herbal Epsom salt.

- Use aromatherapy by lighting scented candles or using a diffuser filled with essential oils to relax the body and lift your mood.

---

137 If your pain pattern is more intense, prolonged, or debilitating than usual, contact your health-care professional.

- Watch videos or podcasts that provide guided imagery and breathing meditations to relax.

- Distract yourself by listening to your favorite music or bilateral music (described in chapter 15), streaming favorite shows, reading, talking with a friend, or cuddling with a pet.

- Use a TENS unit to distract from the pain sensations.

- Keep up with all effective strategies.

When the pain begins subsiding, give yourself points for practicing comforting strategies to minimize the flare-up. Many of my clients try to resume their normal activities too quickly. This often backfires and sets them back into another flare-up. Oftentimes they're anxious about catching up with all the things they've fallen behind on. I have found the best way not to be guilty of this is to slowly reintroduce daily tasks into your days. "Slowly" means "do less than you think you can do."

Moving Forward Post Flare-Up

- Keep up with all effective treatment strategies.

- Avoid all known triggers whenever possible.

- Prioritize rest and sleep.

- Eat a healthy diet and stay hydrated.

- Reduce stress.

- Stretch and keep moving.

The suggested flare-up hacks can be invaluable in improving your quality of life. Remember also that self-compassion, patience, and persistence are important companions in your quest toward improved pain management and overall well-being.

Appendix C

Resources: The World of Apps

In the first decade of the 2000s a revolution burst forth in the health self-management arena with the launch of apps, software programs designed for specific tasks on mobile devices or computers. Suddenly, the market was flooded with them. Each one was uniquely designed to give power to the individual to dramatically improve their health. With the touch of their smartphones, they could tap into the power of tracking their health and well-being markers like never before.

Apps have come a long way in the few short years since they showed up on the scene. When they first arrived, they did simple tasks like counting calories, tracking fitness metrics, and sending medication reminders. Then the creators came up with wearable devices that also tracked heart rate, sleep, and total steps taken.

Before we caught on to that, specialized apps arrived to go further in following particular conditions that required more in-depth support like diabetes, mental health, and pregnancy. Then augmented reality (AR) and virtual reality (VR) joined the revolution to create physical therapy exercises, meditation sessions, and cognitive therapy in a virtual environment.

After that, telemedicine, which we have already explored in this book, emerged. At the time of this writing, artificial intelligence (AI) is now able to analyze data with amazing accuracy. It has proven that it can predict health flare-ups in chronic conditions. The apps also moved into providing the chronic pain patient with the ability to tap into online community, allowing participants to interact with each other.

Designers are currently working on making apps that help people manage their pain at home as an affordable and accessible option in addition to any medical treatments recommended by their health-care professionals. I happen to be partnered with the neuro-wellness company TrainPain, whose innovative neuroplasticity app that retrains the brain to dial down pain sensations was awarded the grand prize by the Academy of Pain Medicine and MIT Hacking Medicine in 2023. To learn more of my adventures with this company, be sure to join me on my social media, where I will be posting updates.[138]

Also on the forefront is redesigning the apps to address accessible issues and to make the offerings more inclusive. Even though the app development is impressive, it doesn't take the place of the need to work with your health-care professional.

If you're interested in exploring this digital frontier that's ever-evolving, I've provided a list of the types of apps my clients have found useful. I didn't name specific brands since the market is rapidly changing.

The list is intended to empower you to explore, compare, and choose an app that best aligns with your specific needs and preferences. Remember, you're an experiment of one, and the app that works for someone else may not be the

---

138 Bonnie Lester (@bonbonlester), "TrainPain presents: Overcoming CRPS," Instagram, October 21, 2023, https://www.instagram.com/p/CyrA2iFPxrD/.

right one for you. Whether you're seeking to track symptoms, find relaxation techniques, build a community, or gather insights, an app can be your ally.

Types of Apps for Pain Management

Pain Tracking

How They Work

It might sound daunting to track your pain, but the great thing about these apps is they are designed to log the event and circumstances with a few taps of the buttons on your phone or tablet. These apps record your pain levels and possible triggers by looking at your activity, energy level, food consumed, and the weather when you experience an increase.

Value

This kind of information aids you in making decisions. The data highlights patterns that are contributing to your discomfort. An app like this might be the key to understanding what you can do to feel better.

Medication Reminder Apps

What They Do

This type of app is uniquely designed to make sure you stay on top of taking your medication to keep your pain manageable. They send timely reminders on your phone or smartwatch. They even remind you when it's time for a refill.

How They Work

The user enters the details of each medication they're taking, including dosage, frequency, and any specific instructions the doctor has given, such as taking with food or keeping the medicine in the refrigerator.

Value

No more worrying about remembering to take what pill when and how. These apps will give you peace of mind and keep you up to date on how consistently you are taking your medications.

Movement and Exercise Apps

What They Do

This type of app is built for people who are concerned about pain management and need exercise and movement to help improve their condition. Think of it like having a virtual trainer on your phone or tablet. These apps provide a wealth of information about the physical pain management approaches. Users can set goals, track progress, and vary routines. Additionally, these apps use reminders, achievement badges, and other gamification techniques to keep users motivated.

How They Work

These apps take users through tailored exercises and physical activities based on personal input and their personal goals. Wearable devices track performance and adjust exercises based on real-time data.

Each exercise is provided with a visual demonstration along with a step-by-step guide. Tips are provided on how to do the exercise correctly. These apps automatically track their progress and suggest routine variations. In addition, the users have access to a library of exercises to aid in their pain management.

Value

Physical activity, when done correctly, can significantly reduce pain. These apps are designed to guide you through how to do exercises and which ones will be most helpful for your condition. Using these apps reduces the risk of injury of going at it solo.

Mindfulness and Meditation Apps

How They Work

They provide tools for beginner to advanced levels of mindfulness training with breathing, walking, and eating. They provide a library of audio/video sessions, including body scans, progressive relaxation, guided imagery, and loving-kindness meditation. Users can customize their selection based on focus, duration, style, and background music.

Value

Meditation and mindfulness apps tap into the ability to reprogram how our brains interpret pain, dialing that down and increasing relaxation. With regular practice, people's quality of sleep increases.

Educational Resources

How They Work

They offer articles, videos, and interactive content about specific pain conditions and their causes, symptoms, and available treatments to help users understand the mechanisms of chronic pain. They are developed and curated by reputable medical institutions and health-care professionals to ensure the information is accurate and up to date. Some of these apps allow users to track their pain levels, triggers, and patterns.

Value

This data educates the user so they can make informed decisions about their condition.

Connect with Others

How They Work

These apps open the door to connect people who are living with chronic pain, providing a social community to share experiences, ask questions, and offer support to one another.

Users post questions, tips, and experiences that others can read and comment on.

Value

These apps provide the ability to talk to others who are suffering from similar conditions.

The Cost of Pain Management Apps

The cost of these apps can vary widely depending on the features they offer. Some offer free basic features to download with premium add-ons for lifetime access or ongoing subscriptions. By checking the app store, you'll find the most up-to-date pricing information for specific apps.

Find Reviews for Health Management Apps

With the continual evolution of apps, it's a good idea to check the latest app reviews, ratings, and recommendations to pick the one that will best suit your health needs.

Ways to gather information to help you pick the right app:

- **Ask health-care professionals:** Consult with health-care providers who may have insights and recommendations into effective pain management apps. Doctors are on the front lines and often receive feedback about various apps from their patients. If you have conditions that might be triggered by apps, it is also a good idea to double-check with your physician before starting with one.

- **App stores:** Visit the site and search for the specific health management app you're interested in. Scroll down to "Ratings and Reviews" to read users' reviews and ratings.

- **App review websites:** These websites and platforms specialize in reviewing and recommending health and wellness apps:

- CNET

- Healthline

- Medical News Today

- PCMag

- Verywell Health

- **Social media:** Search for the app's name on social media platforms like Reddit, Facebook, or Instagram. Users often share their experiences and opinions about apps. Keep in mind when reading the reviews that not everyone will leave a five-star review. Some users may leave an extremely negative review simply to be malicious or because they are a competitor. Be sure to filter out the naysayers who might discourage you from using an app that could be of benefit.

- **YouTube:** Search for video reviews or tutorials about apps in this format. Many content developers and influencers share their experiences and thoughts with pain management apps.

- **Word of mouth:** If family members, friends, or coworkers use pain management apps, ask them for feedback.

Remember, reviews can be subjective, so consider gathering up multiple sources to get a better understanding of an app's strengths and weaknesses before selecting one.

Apps have completely changed the world of chronic pain sufferers. Each app offers something different, but all of them are working to provide sufferers with solutions to some of their struggles. Using these digital tools can make a significant difference in your quality of life.

If an app doesn't work for you, try another. Don't give up. Everyone is different.

Appendix D

The Highways and Byways of Surfing the Web

The ability to surf the web for health information in the privacy of my home was years away when I was diagnosed with CRPS way back in 1986. I never foresaw that I'd have the ability to one day reach for my iPhone to research any topic I wanted.

Being able to access information so readily empowers us to step into a proactive role in the health-related decisions we make. Unfortunately, there are bad actors on the web hawking not only misinformation, but also expensive products backed by unsubstantiated claims.

To help you to evaluate information and feel secure using the web, I'm sharing the following short tutorial.

Evaluate Online Health Information

On the internet, consider:[139]

- **Who runs the site?** Government agencies, medical schools, professional organizations or manufacturers, distributors, self-proclaimed healers, or influencers? Look at the URL (the web address). URLs with .gov, .org, or .edu carry more clout and trustworthiness[140] because these institutions are governed by strict standards and backed with grueling peer-to-peer evaluation.

- **What is the purpose of the site?** Information, promoting opinions, or sales?

- **Who pays for the site?** Consider who funds the website. If it's supported by ads, are they clearly marked as ads? Be on the lookout for overly biased language toward the product or service that the website is selling. More trusted sites are transparent about their affiliations and connections and go through more check-and-balance procedures before publishing their findings.

- **Is the information high quality?** "High quality" means that the articles are backed by legitimate research studies that explain in depth how the research was conducted, and the material has been peer reviewed. If a source is written in a dramatic way, promises cures, or makes claims that sound too good to be true, be wary.[141]

---

139 "How To Evaluate Health Information on the Internet: Questions and Answers," National Institutes of Health, last updated May 4, 2022, https://ods.od.nih.gov/HealthInformation/ How_To_Evaluate_Health_Information_on_the_Internet_Questions_and_Answers.aspx; "Evaluating Health Information," MedlinePlus, accessed March 13, 2024, https://medlineplus.gov/ evaluatinghealthinformation.html.

140 "How to Find Reliable Health Information Online," National Institute on Aging, last updated January 12, 2023, https://www.nia.nih.gov/health/healthy-aging/how-find-reliable-health-information-online.

141 "Evaluating Health Information."

- **Does the site provide details to back up the information's credibility?** Ideally, the site should have a content review process, a selection policy for their content, and an editorial board of health experts. These things are often mentioned on the site's "About Us" page. Information about writers' and researchers' qualifications should also be provided (this is often placed at the bottom of articles).[142]

- **Are there links and references to the sources of the information provided?** Many sites have a separate page dedicated to links and references. Check menus and sidebars for a "Resources" page.

- **Is it up to date?** Always check the date on the material you're reading. An acceptable age of a health article varies depending on the topic and the rate of advancements in the specific field. Fast-evolving topics are dated if they were written three years ago. Topics with slower developments are still relevant if an article was written in the past three to five years. Research your topic to see if it has had recent major breakthroughs.

- **Does the website provide privacy and data use policies?** Do they explain how the website collects, uses, and protects your personal information?

- **Don't stop at one website, post, or forum.** After finding a site you trust, search for other sites that seem legitimate to compare their information or findings. Also read what actual patients have to say about their experiences with various treatments.

On social media, the same considerations apply. Ask where the information comes from, why it is being shared, and who is funding it.

Here's an added bonus on how to find reliable health information from the news and from books.

---

142 "Evaluating Health Information."

In the News

- Does the story say whether the research involved people or animals?[143]

  - **Safety Metric:** Results from human subjects rather than animal studies are typically more reliable for health-related applications. Humans have unique physiology, genetics, and behaviors.[144]

  - **Watch Out For:** Generalized conclusions without explanations of how researchers arrived at their findings are a warning sign that the study might not be trustworthy.

- If the research involved people, how many participants? What was the demographic profile of those who participated in the study?[145]

  - **Safety Metric:** Larger sample sizes and more diverse participants generally produce more accurate results. This is because the larger the sample, the more information will be gleaned regarding unforeseen variables such as side effects.

  - **Watch Out For:** Too small of a group, uncontrolled environment, no direct application, or faulty thinking such as the idea that something is all good or all bad.

- How long was the study?[146]

  - **Safety Metric:** There's no set amount of time that a study must last, but generally speaking, studies that run for years have more robust findings. This gives more time to show results and possible long-term side effects and gives space to explore other variables.

  - **Watch Out For:** Limited studies that make big claims.

143 "Evaluating Health Information."
144 "Problems with Animal Research," American Anti-Vivisection Society, accessed February 21, 2024, https://aavs.org/animals-science/problems-animal-research/.
145 "Evaluating Health Information."
146 "Evaluating Health Information."

- What type of study was it?[147]

  - **Safety Metric:** The best is a randomized placebo-controlled clinical trial. Randomized controlled trials (RCT) are the top standard of research.[148]

  - **Watch Out For:** Anecdotes and observations with limited metrics.

- Were there side effects?

  - **Safety Metric:** Look for reports that list the possible side effects and clearly state the possible known risks.

  - **Watch Out For:** Studies that bury the side effects, don't mention them, or treat them as unimportant.

- Who paid for the research?[149]

  - **Safety Metric:** It's important for studies to be done by organizations that don't directly benefit from the results of the findings.

  - **Watch Out For:** Funding sources that are buried and hard to determine.

- Who's reporting the results?

  - **Safety Metric:** What's the writer's motivation? How reputable are sources, and what is their track record and reputation?

  - **Watch Out For:** Conflict of interest, lack of rigorous testing methods, and lack of staff.

---

147 "Evaluating Health Information."
148 Emily C. Zabor, Alexander M. Kaizer, and Brian P. Hobbs, "Randomized Controlled Trials," *Chest* 158, no. 1S (2020): S79–87, https://doi.org/10.1016/j.chest.2020.03.013.
149 "Evaluating Health Information."

In Books

- How old is the book?[150]

  - **Safety Metric:** Health and medical knowledge rapidly evolves, so oftentimes, books more than three to five years old are dated. That's not to discount the effectiveness of older books based on time-tested health principles.

  - **Watch Out For:** Do a search on the findings to see if they have been refuted or if updated information contradicts them. If you're confronted with contradictory health information, consider seeking guidance from your health-care provider.

- Is the author an expert on the subject?[151]

  - **Safety Metric:** Does the author have a degree in the subject area? Typically, authors with credentials such as MD, PhD, DC, DO, DPT, ND, DNP, or MA in the subject matter are more reliable sources.

  - **Watch Out For:** Misrepresentation of qualifications and making false claims about study outcomes. Always consult the original sources of the information presented.

- Have experts endorsed the book?

  - **Safety Metric:** Having the book endorsed by leading experts and by qualified people in the industry is not a guarantee that the information is credible, but it certainly helps. Most professionals will not risk their name and reputation on something that is not up to their standards.

  - **Watch Out For:** A poorly written book that has inconsistent information, lack of credible sources, and grammatical errors.

---

150   "Evaluating Health Information."
151   "Evaluating Health Information."

If the writer didn't take the time to produce a book of quality, then that's reflective of how they vetted the information they are presenting.

- Does the book list the sources of the content?[152]

  - **Safety Metric:** It's a good sign when the health book provides a source page that lists the origins of the information presented. That gives the reader the ability to double-check the research and the quality of the sources. It is becoming increasingly more important to verify information since the influx of fake research is on the rise.[153]

  - **Watch Out For:** AI-written books and lack of references or citations.

On the day I wrote this, I gave the AI model ChatGPT-4 this prompt:

Question

I'm writing a healing book with the focus audience of patients who are suffering chronic pain. I wanted to get your opinion on whether patients should depend on AI-generated books for health decisions.

ChatGPT-4 Response

When authoring a book aimed at patients with chronic pain, it's important to consider the role and limitations of AI-generated content in health-care decision-making. Here are several reasons why a patient should be cautious about relying solely on AI-generated books for health decisions:

- Accuracy and Reliability: AI-generated content might lack accuracy or provide information based on limited or out of date data.

---

152 "Evaluating Health Information."

153 Bernard Sabel, interview by Ayesha Roscoe, "Fake Studies in Academic Journals May Be More Common Than Previously Thought," *Weekend Edition Sunday*, NPR, May 14, 2023, https://www.npr.org/2023/05/14/1176062276.

- Lack of Context: AI may not fully comprehend the nuances of individuals' health challenges, which leads to generalized recommendations.

- Misinterpretation of Research: AI may misinterpret or over-simplify complex scientific research that can potentially lead to misleading conclusions or recommendations.

- No personalization: AI doesn't base its health recommendations needed on an individual's health history, genetics, and lifestyle.

- Legal and Ethical Issues: Health content generated by AI might inadvertently violate privacy laws or ethical standards if it uses personal health data without proper consent.

- Lack of Accountability: If a problem occurs with the health advice provided by AI, it may be challenging to identify responsibility or hold anyone accountable for the potential harm caused.

- Risk of Misdiagnosis: AI may not have the ability to conduct a comprehensive clinical assessment, potentially leading to incorrect diagnoses or treatment recommendations.[154]

I believe ChatGPT-4's warnings are valid regarding using it as a search engine for up-to-date health information. Though AI can help streamline basic searches on a variety of topics, when it comes to your health, it's important to always consult with your health-care providers.

Navigating the net requires an informed and vigilant approach. By using the tools discussed in this section, you'll be able to discern the most reliable resource materials and gain the ability to make informed decisions about your health and well-being.

---

154 Text generated by ChatGPT, OpenAI, December 11, 2023, https://chat.openai.com/chat.

Additional Resources

When I became a chronic pain sufferer 38 years ago, there were few pain management books that offered information about my condition, but there was a lot of buzz going around about the emerging mind-body connection. This emerging science highlighted how mental and emotional stress can influence physical health. I purchased mind-body books to see if they could help me.

These are three books that I found incredibly helpful and whose information is still relevant today:

1. *The Relaxation Response* by **Herbert Benson:** Dr. Benson, a cardiologist, authored this science-based book to describe the relaxation response that science proved can calm down the body and improve physical and mental health. His relaxation techniques include meditation and deep breathing.

2. *The Relaxation & Stress Reduction Workbook* by **Martha Davis, Elizabeth Robbins Eshelman, and Matthew McKay:** This self-help workbook delves into the impact of stress on both physical and mental well-being. Each chapter offers a different method to calm the body along with on-the-spot exercises to do when you feel

stressed out.

3. ***Seeing with the Mind's Eye: The History, Techniques, and Uses of Visualization* by Michael and Nancy Samuels:** Dr. Samuels is a physician with a background in integrative medicine who focuses on mind-body healing, using elements of art, imagery, and spirituality for improved health. This book focuses on the history and techniques of visualization for restoring the body and mind.

Contemporary Affordable Pain Management Resources

1. *The Pain Management Workbook: Powerful CBT and Mindfulness Skills to Take Control of Pain and Reclaim Your Life* by Rachel Zoffness

2. *The Chronic Pain and Illness Workbook for Teens: CBT and Mindfulness-Based Practices to Turn Down the Volume on Pain* by Rachel Zoffness

Both of these workbooks authored by pain psychologist Dr. Rachel Zoffness offer science-based strategies to turn down the volume of chronic pain so you can get back to living the life you desire.

3. *Back in Control: A Surgeon's Roadmap Out of Chronic Pain* by David Hanscom, MD

Dr. David Hanscom, a renowned spine surgeon, combines cutting-edge neuroscience with practical strategies to help chronic pain sufferers become architects of their own healing in his latest book. His scalpel-free, pill-light approach paves a transformative roadmap for rewiring the brain.

Note: There are many other helpful pain management books, but their cost isn't in alignment with my goal of presenting affordable and accessible options for my readers.

There is another series of books I found helpful by the prominent Australian pain scientist Lorimer Moseley. His groundbreaking work on neuroplasticity is beautifully illustrated in his books. Since they have a high price tag, I'm sharing the titles of some of his free videos on YouTube so you can decide about investing in his books.

1. "Why Things Hurt" (TEDx Talk)

2. "Tame The Beast: It's Time to Rethink Persistent Pain" (an animated description of persistent pain)

Lorimer Moseley is an engaging professional whose special talent of story-telling shines a new light on the latest information about neuroplasticity and chronic pain. His recorded live presentations (available on YouTube) are always engaging and leave the viewer with a sense of hope.

Online Pain Education

RetrainPain (www.retrainpain.org/#lessons): This website provides up-to-date science-based information about pain and offers free online pain education for chronic pain patients and a tuition-based certification program for clinicians.

Lifestyle Resources

Nutrition

1. *For Fork's Sake: A Quick Guide to Healing Yourself and the Planet Through a Plant-Based Diet* **by Rachael Brown:** If you've been tempted to work toward adopting a plant-predominant food program, then this book is for you. The author, Rachael Brown, blends humor with great advice on how to transition to a healthier

and happier whole-food plant-based-focused eating style. This mom, who's lived the experience of changing over from a standard American diet, offers a 10-day guide to help you and your children start feeling better while saving money.

2. **California Balsamic Vinegars:** This company is committed to quality and crafts an amazing array of vinegars that range from sweet fruit balsamic vinegars to savory vinegars that include balsamic vinegar versions of salt-free teriyaki and curry. When my husband transitioned from his meat-and-french-fries-focused diet, these vinegars satisfied his palate, and he devoured any veggie doused in smoked hickory or seven-herb balsamic. My favorite is wild huckleberry, which I used to marinate my fresh fruit that I serve at parties. The company runs cost-saving sales three times a year that you can be alerted to by subscribing to their newsletter. Before using vinegars, double-check if vinegar can impact the absorption or effectiveness of your prescriptions.

Sleep

The Sleep Solution: Why Your Sleep Is Broken and How to Fix It by W. Chris Winter: Dr. W. Chris Winter is a neurologist and sleep medicine specialist whose engaging storytelling helps the reader explore their own sleeping patterns while providing them with tips to improve their sleep hygiene.

My resources list barely scratches the surface of all the helpful information available. It's your turn to explore the world of YouTube and the net to find the hidden gems that will help make a difference in your life.

Acknowledgments

A heartfelt thank you:

To Denise Vivaldo, who, during my interview on her award-winning podcast, *Women Beyond a Certain Age*, put the bug in my ear about authoring a book about my recovery from CRPS.

To Book Launchers for shoring up my grammar and teaching me about book marketing in the 21st century.

To Reverend Doctor Gina Rose Halpern for founding the Chaplaincy Institute of Berkeley in 1999. It was the place where I found my true calling.

To the late Barbara Weiskotten, who assured me that everyone needs a chaplain.

To Dr. Lin for helping me achieve remission from complex regional pain syndrome.

To TrainPain's Dr. Elan Schneider, Laurence Nash, and Jenny Zsiago, who offered me a platform to spread the word about neuroplasticity.

To the Lubarsky family, who loaned me their dog and then entered my life as dear friends.

To the San Rafael High School class of 1970, who confirmed my belief that time and distance could be overcome so we could support one another online during the pandemic—a true representation of the health value of social connections.

To all the past and present chronic pain sufferers I have helped. You continue to bring joy as you report how your life has improved from the first time you chatted with me.

To our three adult kids, Blake, Leia, and Mitchell, who, along with their spouses and kids, have kept the warm glow of connection lit over the years.

To my late parents Arthur and Ruth Sluser, in your wisdom you maintained strong relations with our relatives who to this day provide me with the belief that my words matter.

To my brother Eric and my sister Stacy, whose daily check-ins during the fifteen months of authoring my book lifted my spirits and kept me focused.

To my two exes Kirk and Bob, thank you for our great post-divorce friendships.

And finally, to my techno wizard husband Len, who happily deals with my computer glitches and made this book possible.

Index

LET'S WORK TOGETHER TOWARDS
PAIN RELIEF

Join Bonnie's newsletter to receive the latest scientific-based strategies for pain management directly to your inbox at **bonnielester.com**

Order special bulk purchases for your company, organization, or community by emailing **bonbonlester@gmail.com**

Book Bonnie Lester for speaking events and consultations by emailing **bonbonlester@gmail.com**

CONNECT WITH BONNIE LESTER

 @bonbonlester

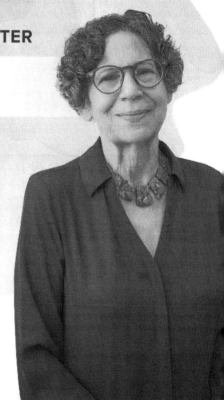

THANK YOU
FOR READING!

If you enjoyed *Unwinding Pain,* please leave a review on Goodreads or on the retailer site where you purchased this book and help me reach more readers like you.

Made in the USA
Columbia, SC
12 September 2024